Cold Wars

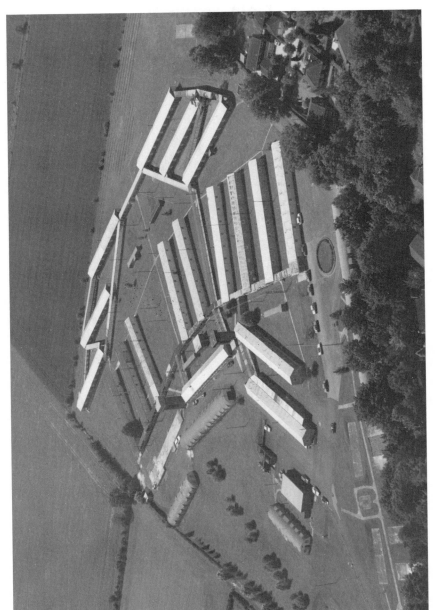

An aerial view of the Common Cold Unit

Cold Wars

The fight against the common cold

DAVID TYRRELL AND MICHAEL FIELDER

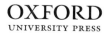

OXFORD
UNIVERSITY PRESS

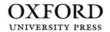

OXFORD
UNIVERSITY PRESS

Great Clarendon Street, Oxford OX2 6DP

Oxford University Press is a department of the University of Oxford.

It furthers the University's objective of excellence in research, scholarship,
and education by publishing worldwide in
Oxford New York
Auckland Bangkok Buenos Aires Cape Town
Chennai Dar es Salaam Delhi Hong Kong Istanbul Karachi
Kolkata Kuala Lumpur Madrid Melbourne Mexico City Mumbai Nairobi
São Paulo Shanghai Taipei Tokyo Toronto

Oxford is a registered trade mark of Oxford University Press
in the UK and in certain other countries

Published in the United States
by Oxford University Press Inc., New York

© David Tyrrell and Michael Fielder, 2002

The moral rights of the authors have been asserted

Database right Oxford University Press (maker)

First published 2002

A catalogue record for this book is available from the British Library

Library of Congress Cataloging in Publication Data
Data available

ISBN 0 19 263285 X

10 9 8 7 6 5 4 3 2 1

Typeset by Integra Software Services Pvt. Ltd, Pondicherry, India
www.integra-india.com
Printed in Great Britain
on acid-free paper by T. J. International Ltd, Padstow

In this age, when cures have been found for so many illnesses, the most widely known complaint of all has defied any attempts to bring it under control. The common cold is everywhere, usually short-lived and rarely fatal. Throughout its history it has been surrounded by fallacies concerning its causes and its effect on our bodies. During the early part of the twentieth century various scientists tried to solve its mysteries but without any notable success. Then, in 1946, the British Medical Research Council decided that the time had come for a more concerted onslaught. The Common Cold Research Unit was brought into being. It was staffed by a brilliant and sometimes eccentric collection of people. And it was destined to make a major contribution to our understanding and treatment of the common cold.

Preface

Much of my life has been spent in the study of colds and influenza. For 33 years I worked at the Common Cold Research Unit (the name was shortened in the 1960s to the Common Cold Unit, or CCU) at Salisbury, arriving there in 1957 and staying until my retirement in 1990. It was then that colleagues, volunteers, and friends suggested that I should write the story of this unique British institution. So I set about preparing an historical account, helped and encouraged by the Twentieth Century History Group of the Wellcome Institute for the History of Medicine. And Oxford University Press was kind enough to express an interest in publishing it.

My retirement turned out to be in name only so that almost 10 years were to pass before I was able to come back to OUP with a first draft. However, its view was that, in this case, a conventional history was not the ideal format and that a book for general readers was a better idea. It repeated an earlier suggestion that it would like to see an explanation of the exciting new medical and scientific ideas on colds and similar diseases that had emerged in the past few decades. It also suggested that I find a partner with experience in writing for both technical and non-technical readers.

I was fortunate to find an ideal collaborator in Michael Fielder, a writer I had known for some years. We decided to do more than just describe what we now know about the causes and treatment of colds. We would outline how the thought of applying science to the study of colds began to emerge from old fashioned theories; how experiments were started on the initiative of some remarkable people; the effect of world events, particularly the world wars, on research; the cooperation of volunteers from the general public; and the dramatic advances in medical and biological science that took place over this period. There were also related subjects to consider, such as the important, and often unforeseen, contributions that work on colds has made to health psychology and a reduction in deaths among children in developing countries.

Throughout the twentieth century there were teams somewhere in the world tackling questions on what causes colds and how to resist them. Their work was not widely reported, being largely written up in specialist journals, so the average person would hear little about it. Those newspapers which did comment from time to time often gave the impression that a cure was just around the corner when it clearly was not. So it has been a case of too little information and much of that misleading. This book has attempted to redress the balance and, hopefully, provide the general reader with a better understanding of the common cold.

The beginning of the twentieth century saw the start of a worldwide movement aimed at using science and experiment to answer specific questions about diseases, rather than making educated guesses based on general ideas about how the body worked. The principles of how to do this were developed in connection with other diseases and then applied to questions about the common cold. The first methods used were derived from the new science of bacteriology and produced a number of confusing possible causes. But in the end meticulous work in New York convinced almost everyone that colds were caused by a virus, even though it was not at all clear what a virus was. Some of the answers were to come by answering the apparently irrelevant question, 'Do bacteria have virus infections?' Although this sounds stumbling and inefficient, science often moves forward in this way. Only rarely do we experience the sudden, dramatic discovery that produces a quantum leap in a particular area.

It would be an attractive idea to describe our advances in knowledge as a series of logically planned and orderly steps from darkness and ignorance to light and understanding. Unfortunately, in our experience, progress rarely occurs like this. Individual brilliance, of course, plays its part, and a very important part, but beyond that it is more often a matter of patient repetition and checking, and being prepared to go on in the face of repeated disappointments. Research workers in more than one field have likened their experience to walking across a darkened room, constantly bumping into various objects. Only later, when eyes adjust to the gloom, can they look back and see exactly how the furniture is arranged. But that is only part of the story. When they switch on the light they discover another door and another darkened room. And the whole process is repeated. Soon they realise that they are in a big house with many rooms, and uncovering all its mysteries will take a very long time.

Enthusiasm for the work is essential. I count myself fortunate to have been part of such an enjoyable and remarkably successful worldwide enterprise. And I was paid for doing it! Throughout I have been driven both by a sense of wonder at the reactions of viruses and the human body and the belief that what is discovered will really help sick people. My hope is that we can convey to the reader some idea of what it feels like to be involved in scientific studies that are so deeply concerned with the health of each one of us.

Looking back on those years of cold research I still wonder why we were given so much official support in the late 1940s. I can only think it was because colds and coughs were regarded as a significant health problem then. Anything which kept people away from work during the war was a serious matter, and much publicity was directed towards reducing the risk of catching colds. Nowadays they seem to be accepted as an inevitable part of everyday life, and children and adults are expected to ignore them as far as possible. Indeed, missing work because of a cold may be regarded as a sign of poor management or poor morale in an employee. Science was seen as the key to the future, and scientists, who had helped so much in winning the war, were expected to start solving peacetime problems in a big way.

Medical research lies at the heart of this story and so, even in a book intended for the general reader, it has been necessary to include the essentials of the science involved. However, we have tried to treat this with a light touch and not allow it to loom large in more than a few chapters. These describe a little of the research work that was undertaken and the trials and frustrations that accompanied this; and then set out to illustrate the mechanics of how colds are contracted, experienced, and eventually overcome. But for those less interested in these aspects there is more than sufficient compensation in those chapters devoted to the history, individual and communal experiences, treatments, psychological implications, and global nature of the common cold.

We have tried to present as broad a picture as possible but, in a publication of this size, a vast amount has had to be omitted. Nor has it been possible to include all the names of the many people who took part in this great enterprise over so many years—not just scientists here and abroad but the numerous people who supported us in so many ways. I hope no one feels offended by this. The CCU was fortunate to have the services of many distinguished scientists, some of them at the outset of their careers and others who were happy to provide us with the benefit of long experience. Some of their names also appear in the Acknowledgements, and some of the missing facts may be found by looking into the Further reading section.

July 2002   David Tyrrell

Acknowledgements

We wish to thank the following for their help:

The Medical Research Council for decades of support of DT and for access to records; The Wellcome Trust for a grant to cover certain expenses; The History of 20th Century Medicine Group of the Wellcome Institute for the History of Medicine for much general stimulation and guidance and in particular Dr Tilli Tansey and Lady Wilkinson (Lise); Sir Christopher Booth for his comments and for reading the book prior to publication; OUP commissioning editors, Susan Harrison and Helen Liepman.

Those who agreed to be interviewed and recorded:

J. Acornley, Dr W. al-Nakib, A. Amos, M. Andrewes, H. Andrews, Dr G. Barrow, Dr A. Beare, Dr S. Beare (Reed), T. Borthwick-Clark, Dr A. Bradburne, P. Bradburne (Ball), P. Brown, K. Callow, Dr E. Clements, Dr N. Clements, Dr N. Dimmock, N. Gee, B. Head, Dr P. Higgins, Dr O. Lidwell, Dr J. Lovelock, Dr E. Lowbury, Dr R. Phillpotts, B. Porterfield (Burch), Dr J. Porterfield, A. Rogers, A. Simms, Dr E. Stott, Dr D. Taylor-Robinson, K. Thompson, A. Thorn, Dr J. Wallace.

Past members of staff and colleagues who wrote letters:

M. Andrews, Dr F. Aoki, J. Bailey, Dr P. Beeson, Dr P. Chapple, Dr D. Chaproniere, Dr J. Craig, Dr K. Dumbell, Dr T. Flewett, Dr J. Gwaltney, E. Jackson, Dr M. Holmes, Dr J. Hotchin, Dr H. Kay, Dr E. Kellner, Dr E. Kilbourne, M. and P. Kuenert, Dr H. Lambert, H. McEwan, Dr J. Mackenzie, Dr T. McNair Scott, Dr T. Matthews, Dr J. Nunn, L. Langford, Dr H. G. Pereira, L. Simon, Dr T. Sommerville, Dr G. Stewart (Walker), Dr J. Wallace.

Previous volunteers and residents, in particular those who wrote, including:

M. Cassie, K. Gatis, H. Grahame, M. Guttridge, J. Haslam, J. Holloway, A. Honeybone, J. Hutchinson, P. and J. Kemp, S. Langridge, V. McLoughlin, A. Mills, K. Nicholson, B. Ollis, R. Parkes, E. Powell, S. Rees, A. Rudd, F. Scott, K. Sellers, D. Simmons, J. Smith, N. Walker, D. Wilkinson.

We obtained access to archive material and early literature through:

The Library of the National Institute for Medical Research and R. Moore (Librarian); the Wellcome Institute Library; the personal papers of Sir Christopher Andrewes (to be archived at the Wellcome Institute); Salisbury Medical Society and Postgraduate Centre Library; and Dr P. Gillam.

The recordings are now kept in the National Sound Archive at the British Library, London and many papers will be found in the Wellcome Library for the History and Understanding of Medicine, London.

Contents

CHAPTER 1

Colds through the centuries

My involvement with the common cold seemed to come about almost by accident, though I suspect that very little in life occurs purely by chance. In 1957 I was running a virus research laboratory in Sheffield. The work was going well and I was looking forward to pursuing my line of research to a successful conclusion. And then an informal message, an even more informal interview, and I found myself transplanted, complete with family, to a remote site in the south of England. I was to run the research programme of the CCU.

It was to be an exciting and challenging project which would take up the major part of my working life. And during its course I found myself following a tortuous trail which led to many blind alleys and disappointments but eventually brought us to the point where we understood a great deal about colds. We discovered many of the organisms that cause them, how they are transmitted, how the body responds to them; we studied the effect of environment on colds and how the mind can also play its part; we took our work into the international arena through our links with World Health Organisation (WHO); and we investigated some of the supposed cold cures that have been promoted, both privately and publicly, over the centuries. But what remains in the mind above everything else in this great adventure is the wonderfully eccentric and very British experiment in the use of human volunteers—in their thousands, eventually, and with their very willing cooperation—in our work on the common cold.

But, of course, I knew nothing of this at the outset and, as I think back over that period, I find it difficult, even now, to explain why I accepted the post. It was a big step for a young scientist and one with a most uncertain future. The challenge that was set before me was to find answers to some of the questions that surrounded the common cold. So, on the one hand, there was the fascination of attacking a problem which had defied a solution for so long and, on the other, the knowledge that better minds than mine had tried and failed. Up to that time no one was quite sure what caused colds or how they were transmitted. If we could throw some light on those mysteries then that was surely worth doing. So I was persuaded.

The common cold has had a remarkably long and successful career, meeting for the most part with a resigned acceptance and little opposition to its progress. Unpleasant but seemingly inevitable, most people have learnt to live with its troublesome symptoms and wait patiently for its passing. The fact that it does pass, in a matter of days and usually without any lasting effects, is probably the reason that earlier generations have not attacked it with more vigour. Adopting a low profile it has insinuated itself into every society throughout history. In fact so low is this profile that the records of early civilisations provide hardly any mention of it. Only in recent centuries do we find any significant reference to colds and their treatment, often bizarre, mostly ineffective, and sometimes painful.

Earliest times

The story of the common cold and the search for its causes and a cure is a fascinating one. When did people first get colds? We don't really know but it was certainly before the dawn of history. People living isolated lives or in small groups remain free of colds but might catch them following contact with the outside world. The solitary, primeval hunter-gatherer may have experienced a life which was nasty, brutish, and short but while on his own he could expect a cold-free existence. It was when he first adopted village life that he probably started suffering from periodic sneezes and sniffles.

Colds were certainly known to the early Egyptians because amongst their ancient hieroglyphics is one for cough and another for coryza or cold. Both have a symbol for something expelled and the second (Fig. 1.1) clearly shows a nose. Records from this period mention a few treatments for coughs and colds, notably in the famous Ebers Papyri. Ebers.763 gives an incantation 'directed against resh which makes ill the seven apertures of the head. This is to be recited in association with the administration of milk of one who has borne a male child and fragrant gum'. Another suggestion 'to drive out catarrh from the nose' is to paint it for four days with galena, dry incense, and honey. It then completes the prescription with a confidence-boosting 'Do it and you will see! Behold it is true!'

The earliest description of a cold that I know of was given in the fifth century BC by Hippocrates, sometimes called the Father of Medicine, who practised and taught on the island of Kos in the Aegean Sea. Remembered chiefly for the 'Hippocratic Oath', which he devised to guide physicians on how to behave ethically, he and his followers taught a form of medicine which was in

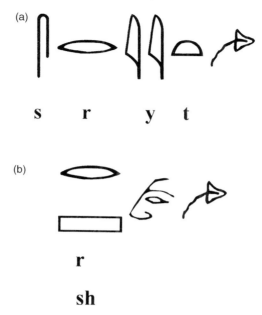

Fig. 1.1 Egyptian Hieroglyphs. (a) A symbol meaning cough. (b) The outline of a nose can be clearly seen together with a symbol for resh, meaning coryza or the discharge of a cold. (From John Nunn.)

advance of their time. In particular they emphasised the importance of carefully observing patients and the results of treatment, and set down their ideas and observations in a series of books. Amongst these was a description of a cold.

In one passage he discusses the effects of 'cold and heat' in the body.

> So long as [they] are present together they are harmless....But when the two principles are separated from each other they then become harmful. The truth of this may be demonstrated by the following consideration of certain signs. An obvious one, and one we have all experienced and continue to do so, is that of the common cold. When we have a running at the nose and there is a discharge from the nostrils the mucus is more acrid than when we are well. It makes the nose swell and renders it hot and inflamed. The fever does not fall when the nose is running, but when the discharge becomes thicker, less acrid, milder and more of its ordinary consistency. Similar changes may be seen as the result of cold alone, but the same observation can be made.

We may not understand or agree with the point he is arguing but there is no doubt that he describes a common cold very much as we know it two and a half thousand years later.

Hippocratic physicians were trying to equate what they saw in patients with what they were taught about the human body and how it worked. They knew that dissected bodies contained fluids (humours). They recognised four: blood in the vessels, black and yellow bile, and phlegm, the clear fluid around the brain. They thought that in health there was a proper balance of these humours and in illness they were unbalanced. For instance an excess of phlegm would leak out through the small holes in the floor of the skull (the cribriform plate) and run out of the nose as rheum and thus cause a cold. If it did not escape it might go down into the joints and cause disease there—hence rheumatism.

Their repertoire of treatments ranged from diet and exercise to preparations of herbs as medicines, and they employed bleeding and cupping to remove 'excess' of blood or clear fluid. The illnesses they treated are described in books such as *Maladies* but, remarkably, do not include cases we would recognise as colds; the nearest being a few cases of angina or sore throat. Either they were not asked to treat colds or else thought them uninteresting or unimportant. But they refer to patients who died from respiratory infections such as pneumonia and pleurisy.

So if people did not go to a doctor with a cold, what did they do? The answer is almost certainly that they treated themselves, using simple remedies handed down to them just as folk-medicines are today. No record has reached us of what these were but we do know that another Greek, Discorides, wrote an extensive treatise on local herbs, how they could be recognised, and what they could be used for. Unfortunately the book did not survive.

The first millennium

Greek medicine and Greek physicians were still highly regarded in Rome several hundred years later. After Hippocrates, by far the most prominent amongst them was a man called Galen, who lived in the second century AD. Born in Pergamum, on the western shores of what is now modern Turkey, he wrote more than a hundred books on medicine and philosophy. So perceptive were his studies of the human body that his ideas continued to influence medical practitioners for nearly 1500 years.

In the first century AD, Celsus, a remarkable Roman physician, wrote a book called *De medicina* (on medicine) and actually described a common cold:

> This closes up the nostrils, renders the voice hoarse, excites a dry cough; in it the saliva is salt, there is ringing in the ears, the blood vessels of the head throb, the urine is turbid. These affections are commonly of short duration, but if neglected may last for a long while.

Amongst the remedies recommended for the common cold was a high quality Italian wine—presumably for the more affluent sufferer.

Pliny the Elder, another remarkable Roman, who wrote on geography and many other topics, also produced a book on herbs based on Discorides. Later he became an admiral in the Roman fleet and, when stationed in the Bay of Naples in AD 79, sailed out to help the inhabitants of Pompeii as Vesuvius pumped ash and lava onto their seaside city. Sadly it cost him his life. But his book and the Greek medical texts survived the break-up of the Roman Empire and the onset of the Dark Ages—notably in the great library at Alexandria in Egypt. Centuries later they were rediscovered by the Moors and, in an Arabic translation, travelled with them as their empire spread outward from the Middle East as far as Spain.

The Renaissance

Preservation of these source books of Greek medicine by the Arabs ensured that they were available for rediscovery when the first medieval faculties of medicine were opened in Europe. There the curriculum consisted largely of learning the works of Galen, though they were over a thousand years old by then. The herbals were also taken up and translated into local languages. And information about northern plants was added to the ancient beliefs about how to use them. As a result the names of old herbalists like Culpepper have survived right up to the present day. And their opinions are quoted by folk who little realise that their ideas originated in the eastern Mediterranean in the fifth century BC.

Northern Europeans certainly had ideas of their own about diseases and their treatment before the classical learning was brought up from the south, but we know little about them. The scholar Charles Singer, writing in 1928, concluded that the Saxons and Normans thought they were due to spirits or arrows flying through the air, and were countered by reciting special spells or incantations.

Thomas Linacre (1460–1524) and his contemporaries at the newly founded Royal College of Physicians of London were excited by the rediscovery of classical learning. But what this offered was a medical art which had hardly advanced since Roman times, albeit far ahead of the old Norse and Saxon superstitions. Thus it included the foundations of botany, chemistry, and pharmacology designed to teach physicians and apothecaries how to recognise and prepare plants, and then to use them as medicines.

It was customary in many houses of the seventeenth and later centuries to keep 'receipt books'. The name refers to drugs or medicines made to a

(a)

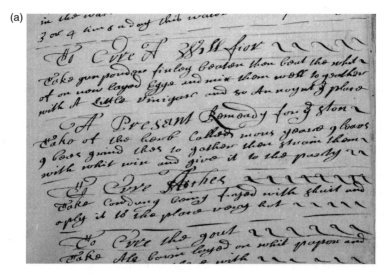

(b)

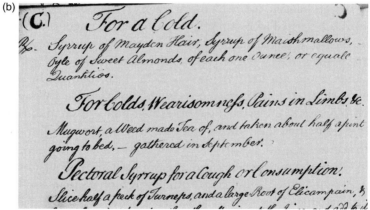

Fig. 1.2 Examples of remedies described in household receipt books. For centuries preparations like these were probably the chief means of treating colds and other ailments in Britain. (a) An extract from Madam Jane Harriott's book begun in 1687. It shows what an extraordinary variety of conditions and recipes such books contained. Her handwriting may be difficult to read and so the transcription below is provided by Anne Young.

To cure a willfior (*wild fire — probably erysypelis*) take gunpowder finely beaten then beat the white of a new layed egg and mix them together with a little vinegar and so annoynt the place.

A present remedy for the stone take of the herb called mouse ears 9 leaves, 9 bees, bring these together then strain them with white wine and give it to the party.

To cure aches take cow dung being fried with suet and apply it the place very hot.

To cure the gout take ale barm (yeast) laid on white paper and lay the place there with.

(b) An extract from Elizabeth Dixon's book begun in 1772. This is indexed and under 'C' has a number of recommended treatments for colds. (From the collection of Anne Young. Photos by John Young.)

particular recipe, rather like the recipe books of favourite dishes kept by the modern housewife. In those days they contained remedies for a range of human and animal diseases, written out in a variety of hands and added to year by year. Some examples of cold remedies are shown in Fig. 1.2. If a family member or servant had a cold the lady of the house would follow instructions in the receipt book to provide them with a drink or inhalation, using materials kept in the house or brought in from the garden or surrounding countryside.

These books give little idea of what sort of disease process they thought they were treating. Phrases such as 'falling down' suggest the Greek idea of a humour descending into the nose. In other cases they mention a 'hot' remedy, suggesting that, in their view, they had a 'cold' disease which should be treated by an 'opposite'. Probably many of them, particularly the patients, were practical and pragmatic and were satisfied if they felt better or more comfortable after the treatment. For example a hot sweet drink would relieve a sore throat, whilst a mild sedative or opiate would have been good for sleeplessness and discomfort. And a rest in bed with a light diet would certainly have been a good prescription for someone with general, influenza-like symptoms.

Primitive physick

The physicians of the eighteenth century tried to base their practice on the scientific knowledge of the day. They called it 'philosophy', and it reflected the advances in medicine that had been made in the past two centuries—the first for about a thousand years. For instance Vesalius dissected the human body in the sixteenth century and found that it was not as Galen had said; and in 1628 Harvey showed that blood circulated through the heart and blood vessels. But in spite of these discoveries ancient treatments such as cupping and bleeding were still widely used.

Some of the remedies must have seemed quite logical to those who believed that diseases were due to spirits and demons entering the body. Such intruders had to be driven out. Examples of this have been recorded in more recent times. Relieve a cough by coughing into the mouth of a frog was one solution on offer. Apparently, in the spring when respiratory diseases were common, the Pueblo Indians of North America had a village event in which 'disease and witches are whipped away with eagle plumes'. At the end of the night 'the head doctor thanks everyone and hopes that all sickness has been dispelled and all witches dispersed'.

Herbs and folk medicines

Page 1373 Juniper Tree—which is described as hot and dry

'The fume and smoke of the gum doth stay flegmatic humours that distill out of the head, and stoppeth the rheume.'

Page 1086 Nigella—possibly our Love-in-a-mist

The seed dried powdered and 'wrapped in...lawne' 'cureth all mucus, catarrhes, rheumes and the pox...being often smelled into from day to day and made warm at the fire when it is used.'

Page 400 Wilde Poppie

'...the knobs or heads, which doe specially prevail to moove sleepe, and to stay and repress distillations or rheums' and he says is more gentle than opium.

Pages 369 and 359 Tabaco or Henbane of Peru

'dried leaves...taken in a pipe and suckt into the stomacke and thrust forth against the nostrils against the pains of the head, rheumes aches in any part of the body...'

Page 813 Mountain Coltsfoot

'A decoction made of the greene leaves and roots, or else a syrup there-of, is good for the cough that precedeth of a thin rheume.'

Entries from John Gerard's herbal of 1633 give some idea of what an apothecary might prepare for someone with a cold or some such problem.

It is not surprising that people resorted to their own remedies. The medical profession had a somewhat tarnished image. It was criticised for its high charges and mistrusted because of doubt surrounding the remedies it used. These were kept secret and could be harmful, either because their full effects were not understood or because they might be made up inaccurately or from impure ingredients.

One of the people who addressed these problems was, surprisingly, John Wesley. Well known as a talented linguist and preacher, he started as a priest of the Church of England, served as a missionary in the American colonies, and founded the Methodist Church when he returned to England. But he also wrote a book entitled *Primitive physick or an easy and natural method of curing most diseases* because he believed that simple means would maintain and restore health and avoid recourse to expensive and harmful physicians and apothecaries. He may have had more experience than usual from his contacts with Native Americans, though one suspects that he also drew on other sources. He advised a healthy lifestyle—taking regular daily exercise and

disease pattern could be repeated. For some this pointed to the cause being a 'poison' that could replicate itself. But no one applied this idea to colds.

Lawrence considered that the culprit might be something in the air. And others, more specifically, blamed the foul air in the filthy streets of London and other burgeoning cities for the high death rate there. It provoked the founding of the Hygienic Movement to clean up the cities, and this had some success.

In the 1850s John Snow, who became president of the Medical Society, showed that cholera was transmitted through drinking the water in London, and Florence Nightingale showed what could be done in the army through cleaning and disinfection. Ten years later W. Austin, an army doctor, in a text-book *The science and practice of medicine*, advocated the examination of urine chemically, and the use of thermometer, microscope, and stethoscope. He also placed a high value on clinical observation, pointing out that smallpox begets smallpox just as cholera begets cholera, and that there could be 'poisons' in the patients that could propagate themselves and spread from person to person.

The idea of living infectious agents was still unpopular although, in 1840 in Germany, F. G. J. Henle had argued for their existence and set out his theories (later known as the Koch—Henle postulates), which would provide conclusive proof that a cause for disease had been found. These stated that the agent would be found in sick people and not in healthy subjects; that it could be propagated in the laboratory; that it would produce the disease when inoculated into a susceptible animal; and that it could then be recovered again and grown in pure culture.

In the 1850s and 1860s Louis Pasteur in France discovered that chemical changes in wine and milk were due to microbes and, by careful experimentation, showed that the bacteria and yeasts in fermenting fluids were essential for the process. Furthermore, these did not develop spontaneously but were introduced; and if they were kept out or killed then the fluids stayed sterile. He also showed that two diseases of silkworms were due to infection with microbes. This led him to develop a general germ theory concerning the transmission and cause of diseases in both animals and humans. Pasteur then set out to prove the validity of his theory. First he demonstrated how animals could be protected against infection by injecting them with vaccines prepared from germs grown in his laboratory. Then, in a public display, he showed how his vaccine would protect sheep from a later injection of live anthrax bacteria. He also developed vaccines against chicken cholera and rabies.

The English surgeon, Joseph Lister, seized on his ideas to develop and spread the idea of antiseptic surgery. He accepted the theory that sepsis could be caused by airborne infection and introduced rules of hygiene which brought a dramatic reduction in deaths following surgical operations. In his own operating theatre, using carbolic acid as an antiseptic, these deaths fell from 40% to 15%.

In Germany Robert Koch, formerly a student of Henle, began his medical career in a country practice but then took an interest in research. He wanted to find the cause of tuberculosis. Like Pasteur he introduced improvements in research techniques: he found a way to stain the tubercle bacillus so that it could be readily observed under the microscope; developed better sterilising methods using high pressure steam; and grew organisms on the surface of jellies, where each one formed a single colony and then could be counted and purified. With these methods he was able to detect a characteristic bacillus in diseased tissues, grow it in the laboratory in pure culture, and then reproduce the disease by injecting it into guinea pigs—in which he again found the bacilli. This was research work of the highest standard and it was rightly acclaimed throughout the world. Later, when travelling to Africa, he discovered the bacterium that causes cholera.

These successes made people realise there might be other diseases that were due to specific microbes and which might be prevented by vaccination.

More than just bugs

The work of Koch and others demonstrated that there were microscopic living organisms that could infect people and cause diseases; and it was recognised that there were methods, such as good hygiene, heat treatment, and antiseptics that could reduce the incidences of such diseases. But little was known about these organisms, other than that they existed. Their variety, size, structure, and effect on our bodies were mysteries which would be solved only after painstaking research throughout much of the twentieth century; and even now there are many more secrets still to be unravelled.

Many people may think of these infectious agents simply as bugs or germs, without distinguishing much between them, but we now know that there are a number of well-defined groups and, within these, further subgroups, each of which is responsible for a specific type of disease. Quite a number can be lumped under the general heading of microbes, and amongst these we would include protozoa, fungi, and bacteria.

Protozoa are single-celled animals which can invade the body and cause disease, malaria being an example. Certain fungi infect surfaces, causing thrush and ringworm, and some produce effects which are more deep-seated. Both of these are life forms that have their genes inside the cell nucleus and are called eukaryotes, a group which contains most organisms other than bacteria. But bacteria are more frequent causes of infection, though generally smaller and more primitive creatures. Their genes are not contained in a nucleus and they are known as prokaryotes. These come in a variety of shapes, sizes, and chemical composition, and they are responsible for some of our major diseases such as tuberculosis and cholera. Boils and other forms of sepsis can also be laid at their door.

Naturally, when the scientific study of colds began it was supposed that they were the result of some form of bacterial attack. The problem for the early researchers was that they could not detect anything that could be identified as a possible single cause. All the organisms so far mentioned could be seen with a light microscope; would grow in non-living media, soups, and jellies; produce changes visible to the naked eye; and could be removed from a solution by passing it through a fine filter. But early researchers found that diseases might still be transmitted with a liquid that had passed through filters that would hold back bacteria. It was the same with a number of other infectious diseases where the tissues and secretions contained no protozoa, fungi, or bacteria. Clearly they were faced with extremely small, submicroscopic particles. And so they called them filter-passing viruses, *virus* being the Latin for poison. But they had to wait for much greater levels of magnification before they could see what it was they had so named. Later they were to find that size was not the only distinguishing characteristic of these strange agents of infection. There were hundreds of different types, structurally primitive but clever; but could they be described as a life form? It was to be a world of bewildering complexity.

New theories and old ideas

Suggestions during the 1890s that at least some colds might be infectious led to researchers using the new bacteriological methods to look for bacteria in the nose of cold sufferers, and a few papers were published. However, the results were confusing because several different types of bacteria were found and the types differed from case to case. Furthermore, the noses and throats of healthy people also contained similar bacteria.

Nevertheless bacteriologists thought they might help patients by vaccinating them. So they grew bacteria from the nose and throat and killed them with heat. They then made up injections of accurately measured numbers of organisms of several types and gave the patient a series of injections. The reports, published in the early 1900s, usually failed to say clearly what happened. But some claimed good results, which probably means that the patient had no colds for the next few months. The methods for clinically testing the vaccines were quite inadequate, and years were to elapse before satisfactory procedures were established. But many people thought that such vaccines were really useful and they were widely discussed and still prescribed in the 1950s, a full half-century later.

Old ideas on the causes of colds were widely believed in the first half of the twentieth century, modified to some extent by the growing science of physiology that had developed steadily from the previous century. Many medical authors, who said that colds were due to chilling, now explained them as due to the chill 'disturbing neurological regulation', whatever that was. A well known physiologist, Leonard Hill, so convinced that colds were due to people going from overheated rooms into the cold outside, said the illnesses should really be called 'fug'. He also taught that regular cold baths protected against the disease, much as Wesley and others had done in the eighteenth century. He and others continued teaching this into the 1920s, and generations of boarding-school pupils probably suffered from his doctrines when they were made to take cold showers every morning.

But other theories were popular. The bowel, known to be full of bacteria, was called the 'sewer of the body' and toxins from these bacteria were blamed for many ills. In some cases the colon was removed, but for problems like colds regular colonic irrigation was proposed. A Dr Tyrrell of New York (no known relative) recommended his own patented 'Cascade' apparatus for the purpose, and his book on its use went to at least 180 editions! I suspect that while all these ideas were being promoted most individuals ignored medical opinions and treatments. They might scold their children for coming home with wet feet but would treat colds with simple drinks and medicines, made up at home or by a local chemist, followed by a bath and early bed.

The birth of virology

It was on the eve of the First World War that the virus theory of the common cold was given substance through some remarkable work being carried out in Germany. Leipzig was the setting for these experiments. An important city for centuries, it lay at the centre of rich farmland and had grown wealthy through trade and industry. Many important roads ran through it and the first German railway had its terminus there. Rich in medieval buildings and historical associations: J. S. Bach, and later Mendelssohn, performed, taught, and composed there; Goethe and Wagner were students at the town's ancient university; and a late-nineteenth century graduate from the medical school, Paul Ehrlich, later to win the 1908 Nobel Prize for medicine, founded the science of specific immunity and began the search for specific drugs against infectious organisms.

The Faculty of Medicine there was amongst the earliest of its kind to be established in Europe. Founded in 1415 it had kept pace with advances in medical knowledge, leading to the introduction of an Institute of Hygiene in 1878, only the third in Europe. Developed as a separate unit it was, by 1906, the largest in Germany. And it was here that a certain Professor W. Kruse, claimed to be the most high-profile hygienist of his time, conducted research and presented regular courses in bacteriology.

Walter Kruse (born 1864) was trained in the methods of Koch, and in 1898 identified the dysentery bacillus (discovered independently by Shiga in Japan). He was a prolific researcher and writer with varied interests, including community health, and in 1907 published a massive textbook on general bacteriology. He was appointed professor in 1913.

Kruse had followed the literature on the cultivation of bacteria such as pneumococci, micrococci, and haemophilus and acknowledged that they appeared to be the cause of colds when they were found in large numbers in catarrhal secretions. In research on pneumococci he concluded that bacteria could only account for occasional colds or for small epidemics and not for most cases. He was also aware of the 'invisible' and filterable viruses which had been talked about during the previous 20 years: he mentions a plant virus and five animal viruses and listed 10 human viruses (not all would now be included), ending with infantile paralysis. The virus for this had been demonstrated in 1909 in Germany, France, and the USA by inoculating monkeys.

In January 1914 his assistant, Dr Hilger, had a cold and Kruse describes how they took full advantage of the opportunity which this presented.

> Secretion blown from his nose was diluted 15-fold in physiological salt solution, filtered through a small Berkfeld filter and a few drops were placed in the noses of 12 colleagues from the Institute. The effectiveness of the filter was determined by cultures. This first experiment resulted in four of the inoculated persons (33%) having a cold after an incubation period of 1–3 days.

When Hilger had another cold on 15 June, Kruse tried a larger experiment, inoculating 36 of his students, 15 of whom developed colds. This compared with 29 students and seven staff who had refused inoculation, amongst whom there was only one cold with an incubation period of one day. He concluded that 'it is highly likely that the cause of at least one form of coughs and colds belongs to the group of invisible or filterable germs. Perhaps it is the most usual form of this disease.' He added that these early results were published so

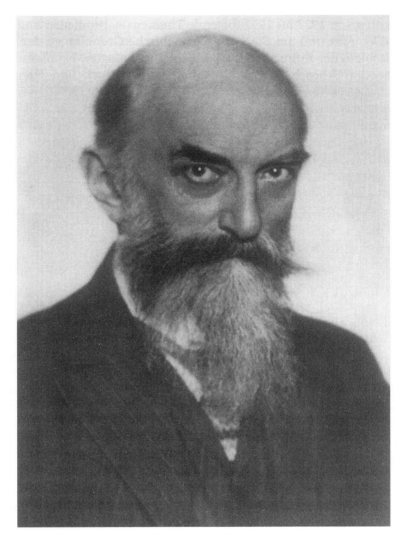

Fig. 1.3 Professor W. Kruse. (From the University of Leipzig.)

that other researchers could take part in the study, and recommended that they investigate other illnesses of the mucous membranes, such as sore throat (angina) and influenza, in a similar way because 'these illnesses do not seem to me in any way adequately explained'.

Kruse reported this work to a meeting of the Leipzig Medical Society on 23 June, only eight days after the second set of inoculations. It was published as a report, and therefore without full references to the literature, on 14 July.

Within weeks Europe was plunged into the First World War and it is sad, but not surprising, that the work was not followed up in Leipzig. The medical school became involved in the care of the sick and wounded and Kruse was concerned with producing and testing cholera and typhoid vaccines. He probably realised the importance of his detection of a cold virus, but it seems as though the practical needs of the war and then the urge to do something to improve the health of society, went to the top of his agenda, and it was left to others to follow it up.

Cold confusion

Teachers of what are seen as complex subjects like science have a difficult job. In dealing with a particular development they may well simplify matters by presenting just the main facts, leaving out any reference to how they were discovered, what theories were followed and found to be wrong, and how long it all took. The complexities of the affair are lost and students then see the whole process as a simple progression towards the correct answer. It all looks so straightforward, even obvious, and, with the benefit of hindsight and the certainty of youth, they may conclude that some of those early investigators were very stupid not to realise that the theories of the day, to which they clung so determinedly, were quite wrong. But those involved in this kind of work know that such things can often be established only when years of careful research have added new ideas and new techniques to the knowledge of the time.

There are many examples of what seem to us quite irrational theories which were accepted at the time they were proposed. Phlogiston is a good example. This was thought to be a substance of negative weight which was released when things burned. It was believed that combustible materials, like wood, were composed of wood ash and phlogiston and that, when they burned, phlogiston flew off in the flame leaving the ash behind. However, early chemists showed that when materials such as metals were burned or corroded they increased in weight, due to the newly discovered element, oxygen, being taken up.

We can see how slow and difficult progress can be as we trace the story of colds. The early belief that such illnesses were due to evil spirits eventually gave way to more rational, but still erroneous, explanations involving body humours and the relationship between climate and people's health. It was at least two thousand years before these ideas were seriously challenged by observation and experiment. Not until the time of Galileo was it shown that the body is always losing fluids into the air.

As we have seen, by the eighteenth century it was reasonable to suggest that if conditions forced changes on the circulation and perspiration then fluid would emerge some other way—through the nose. So ideas about colds were shifted.

It is strange that people did not seem to grasp the idea of infections before the nineteenth century. The evidence was there, long before. During the Black Death in the fourteenth century some cities in southern Europe noticed that if travellers from affected areas stayed outside the town for 40 days they would not transmit the disease when they came in, and so they introduced the idea of, and word for, 'quarantine'. We must assume that in the colds of those days they could not recognise a clear line of spread from one person to another; and if they did they would not understand what it was that passed between them. Antony van Leuwenhoek, the seventeenth-century Dutch investigator, had seen microbes or 'animalcules' years before this, but nobody recognised that these might invade people and make them sick. And because colds often occur in the autumn it was easier to explain them as being due to the season.

Discoveries began to come thick and fast as new laboratory methods were applied to the problem. When Pasteur and Koch founded the science of bacteriology in the mid-nineteenth century, it created a lot of public interest. By the turn of the century people had started to grow bacteria from colds and the first virus infections of plants and animals had been discovered. But popular and medical writing still assumed that colds were usually due to chills.

It seems likely that Walter Kruse did something ahead of his time. He had shown that bacteria caused dysentery, but his study of respiratory diseases convinced him that bacteria were not the causes of most colds. He also took up the idea that viruses caused some diseases of man which were not obviously infectious (like poliomyelitis), and in 1914 did his special experiments in volunteers. In this case he used humans instead of monkeys, presumably because they were most likely to be susceptible to the possible virus and, as it was a mild illness, unlikely to come to any harm. But in spite of his clear results they were not widely understood or accepted generally, and many years of confusion and contradiction followed. He may have been lucky that his results turned out so well since the techniques still needed to be improved. But some so-called improvements were to hinder progress.

Culture shock

Next to study the problem was George B. Foster Jr in the USA. In 1917 he reported experiments he had done on American soldier volunteers which seemed to confirm the results of Kruse, though some of his volunteers had symptoms within six hours of inoculation, which seems unlikely. He also claimed that he had cultured the virus in the test tube. He used a method developed and promoted by a well-known Japanese scientist, Hideyo Noguchi, working on poliomyelitis at the Rockefeller Institute in New York. This was the first institute devoted to biomedical research to be founded in the USA, and Noguchi worked there with the outstanding biologist and director of the institute, Dr Simon Flexner, on a variety of infectious diseases—in the end for over a quarter of a century.

Noguchi claimed that he had grown the poliomyelitis virus in a culture medium of chopped tissue under an oily overlay. His method involved chopping up rabbit kidney and placing it in test tubes containing human ascitic fluid and sealed with a layer of liquid paraffin. These tubes were inoculated with filtered, infectious material. Some days later small particles of a variety of sizes and shapes appeared in the fluid and he believed that these were virus particles, or clumps of them. He said he could confirm this because he had inoculated the fluid into animals and reproduced the original disease. Though some researchers doubted his claims, the institute was highly regarded and he was generally believed.

This all seemed very promising, but others tried to repeat the experiments with cold materials over the next few years, some managing to produce colds with nasal secretions while some could not. Some filter-passing, anaerobic bacteria were found in cultures and nasal material, and some thought these were the cause of colds. Others did not.

Some years later the problems were tackled systematically and thoroughly by an outstanding microbiological research group at the College of Physicians and Surgeons, the medical school of Columbia University in New York City. The man leading them was Dr Alphonse Dochez. Born in California, Dochez had received his medical training at Johns Hopkins University in Baltimore, Maryland. Johns Hopkins had strong links with the Rockefeller Institute in New York at that time and it was there that he went to do laboratory research on bacteriology, later moving to Columbia University. He recognised the first of the serotypes of pneumococci, the bacteria associated with pneumonia, and by 1917 had published a major monograph on treatment of the disease with antipneumococcal serum. He also worked on the serotypes of streptococci and showed that they caused scarlet fever. He was thus in the third phase of a life of research on human infections when he started his studies on common colds in the 1920s. Later he became a professor of Surgical and Medical Research.

Dochez began by studying five of his laboratory staff through the winter of 1925–26. Noses and throats were cultured regularly and records kept of when they got colds. They found that the type and amount of bacteria changed from time to time, but these changes did not coincide with the onset of colds. In fact these might be accompanied by fewer bacteria. Their conclusion was that, contrary to the view held by many at the time, colds could not be caused by bacterial infection.

Their next question was whether filter-passing, anaerobic bacteria caused colds. They discovered that about 70% of people had these strange bacteria, regardless of whether they had colds or not; the type of organism grown from healthy people seemed to be the same as that from people with colds; and, as in the previous study, the number of organisms seemed to be less when their subjects caught a cold. It was clear that they were part of the resident bacteria of the normal human nose and throat and did not cause colds in animals or humans. In the end the flaws in Noguchi's methods and conclusions were generally recognised. But they had an adverse effect on common cold research for over 20 years.

Cold virus research begins in earnest

Dochez now decided to look more closely at those strange, submicroscopic particles highlighted by Kruse and try to answer the question, 'Can a virus cause a cold?' And he thought that chimpanzees might help them find an answer. Zoos claimed that chimpanzees were known to catch colds from their keepers, so Dochez's group kept a number of these animals in isolation rooms and studied their responses to infection. It was found that, under normal circumstances, they remained free from illness; but they developed colds very much like those of human beings after they were inoculated with bacteria-free filtrates of nasal secretions from people with colds. They did not catch colds through material transferred from normal people even though they contained filter-passing anaerobes; but they did get colds from secretions that had been strictly filtered and did not contain these organisms.

To complete the studies they did similar experiments on humans isolated in the same strict way. But now they had to cope with the intelligence and enthusiasm of their new 'guinea pigs'. These 'experimental animals' would tend to report cold symptoms if they thought they had been given cold virus. Dochez and his colleagues overcame this problem by inoculating them several times over several days but without telling them whether this was with real filtrates or with a dummy. The volunteers, realising they would appear foolish if they reported a cold after being given a harmless fluid, cut out their over-enthusiastic claims. These precautions were necessary because it was thought that some initial experiments had been flawed in this way, resulting in some implausibly short incubation periods.

Dochez's results had a significant impact on medical science, and the common cold problem was exciting more interest than ever before. It was now clear that colds could be produced by bacteria-free filtrates of nasal fluids and could be passed from volunteer to volunteer. It was also recognised that filter-passing anaerobes existed but did not cause colds. Another research group at the Johns Hopkins Hospital in Baltimore, Maryland had begun experiments with young women as volunteers. These were conducted in the summer, when there would not be many natural colds, and, once again, they showed that colds could be produced by carefully filtered nasal fluids and concluded they were due to a virus. The work of Dochez and his colleagues was now confirmed and could be included in medical textbooks. At last, it was understood that there really was a common cold virus.

But if many now believed that viruses caused colds, the idea was still a long way from being universally accepted. In the following year, 1932, Drs David and Robert Thomson were able to publish *The common cold*, their comprehensive review of literature on the common cold up to that date, which still promoted the view that colds were caused by bacterial infection. Yet almost 20 years had passed since Kruse's conclusive experiment contradicting this. The book ran to some 700 pages, with a passing reference to the 'virus theory' in only 12 of them; which shows how difficult it can be to interpret contradictory results and to reach firm conclusions with imperfect techniques. It also shows that massive learning and detailed knowledge do not inevitably lead us to the truth.

Whilst this was going on in New York there were scientists in Britain who had reached similar conclusions concerning the importance of studying these potential causes of such serious illnesses. In 1918 and 1919 more people died of influenza than were killed in the 1914–18 war, and common respiratory diseases were perceived as interfering with the economy and education. Some thought these diseases were due to viruses, but nobody could prove it. Others said that viruses caused cancer. Nobody knew much about what viruses were or how to test for them. So the newly formed Medical Research Council (MRC) in Britain decided, in the 1920s, that it would promote work on these mysterious organisms. And it was prepared to be opportunistic about it, taking advantage of an offer of funds to develop a vaccine against dog distemper.

The MRC looked for individuals with talent and flair whom it could support to find out all they could about viruses, the intention being that they would study individual viruses. This seemed an essential first stage if it was going to investigate infections more effectively. The MRC therefore appointed a few people to work in this field at the new National Institute for Medical Research (NIMR) in London. One of the key people supported at this stage was a young physician called Christopher Andrewes.

A man of many parts

Dr (later Sir) Christopher Andrewes was a particularly lively medical scientist who trained in clinical medicine at St Bartholomew's Hospital in London but had developed a liking for laboratory work and an enthusiasm for natural history. His father was a pathologist who had worked on influenza but the son began his research career hunting for tumour viruses at the NIMR and then, while at the Rockefeller Institute in New York, spent two years looking for viruses in rheumatism. In the process he showed how viruses could be grown in the primitive tissue culture of the day. It was here he concluded that viruses only grew when living cells were present, confirming the view that there could be no live cells in tissue suffocated by a layer of oil in a Noguchi-type culture.

In 1931 a chance meeting took place which was to have a profound effect on cold research in Britain. Andrewes was stuck in New York waiting until his father, who had suffered a stroke while on a visit to the USA, had recovered sufficiently to be accompanied back to Britain. In order to fill his time more profitably young Andrewes went to visit various individuals whom he had come to know while at the Rockefeller Institute a few years earlier. Amongst these was Alphonse Dochez.

Andrewes' visit took place whilst Dochez and his colleagues were carrying out their experiments with young chimpanzees and humans: inoculating them with bacteria-free filtrates of nasal secretions from people with colds and producing typical colds. He saw the chimpanzees in their sterile isolation rooms, tended by people who were masked, gloved, and gowned as for a surgical operation. And he recognised the significance of what they were achieving. Andrewes was fascinated by the whole project and gleaned as much information as he could during his visit. He had found fault with almost all the previous experiments of this type, but this very conclusive evidence persuaded him that colds really could be due to a virus. He determined to follow up these studies as soon as he returned to Britain.

Inevitably, as he was leaving Dochez's laboratory, there occurred one further query in his ever-inquiring mind. 'What do the chimps do when you leave the

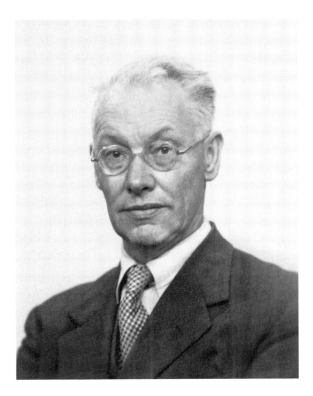

Fig. 1.4 Dr (later Sir) Christopher Andrewes. (From the National Institute for Medical Research London.)

room?' He was told that one of the research team had already attempted to find this out, to discover that a similar question had obviously occurred to the inquisitive anthropoids. When he looked through the keyhole it was to see a brown eye peering back at him!

When Andrewes was back in England he wrote a memorandum, dated 20 August 1931, to the Director of the NIMR Dr (later Sir) Henry Dale. In this he agreed with the preliminary findings of Dochez, but was not so happy with the claim that they had grown the virus in 'hashed chick embryo' tissue. Viruses only grew in tissue of susceptible animals, he believed, but admitted that embryo tissue might be different. He also pointed out that 'the use of living cells in an anaerobic medium is obviously irrational'. The anaerobic medium was used because of the strong belief of Dochez's assistant that, as this helped the virus to survive in the refrigerator or at room temperature, it would also help it to grow.

By then it was widely thought that viruses would multiply only in living cells—and, in the conditions used, all cells would die within a day, as Dochez's group actually showed. Thus Andrewes got Dochez to agree that 'the virus will grow either aerobically in chicken cells or anaerobically without chicken cells'. He then set out a list of exciting experiments that could be done if the virus could be grown and detected in these cultures, followed by a section on 'organisation of volunteers'. There was no prospect of getting a suitable hospital building as they had in New York, but they could use larger numbers of volunteers and dispense with isolation. He admitted that natural colds could affect them and might confuse the results, but he probably saw no alternative at the time. Students and the unemployed were his suggestion for the people to use—so there would be 'no expenses'. Dale's handwritten note altered this to 'relatively small' and criticised the idea of recruiting from the unemployed. Andrewes suggested a compromise scheme:

> It might be possible to rent a house and isolate volunteers in a room in that. The difficulties would be considerable. It would be expensive to furnish and... hard to sterilise between experiments. It would be necessary to have a cook-housekeeper, a resident medical officer—a recently qualified man would do—to observe symptoms and keep discipline—and possibly a housemaid as well...It would be convenient to have the house at Hampstead, but it might be better to have it further out of town and to allow the prisoners out on parole for walks. Possibly volunteers would come more readily if they could be isolated in twos instead of in ones.

He recognised that working on volunteers without isolation would produce inconclusive results. And that spurred his imagination to dream of how rigorous experiments could be done without going to the lengths he had seen in New York. But what is so fascinating is that this reads like a specification for the CCU—15 years ahead of its time.

Cheaper than chimps

Unfortunately Andrewes return coincided with the Great Depression, MRC staff had suffered a salary cut, and money was in short supply. He was offered about £200 to pay for a researcher to help him over a period of six months. Clearly there was not a hope of following up the Dochez experiments using chimpanzees and strictly isolated rooms as provided in the USA. Something cheaper was needed.

Andrewes solved the problem by recruiting students instead. Addressing a meeting of pre-clinical students at St Bartholomew's Hospital in his sparkling and eccentric style, he couched his request in irresistible terms. 'We cannot get hold of any chimpanzees and the next best thing to a chimpanzee is a Bart's student.' Despite this remark, or possibly because of it, 100 students were immediately enrolled.

They may have been 'cheaper than chimps', as he put it, but the problem was that they could not be isolated like chimpanzees—they had to continue their studies. This made it impossible to get really 'clean' results since no one could be certain that any colds caught by the student volunteers resulted from the nose drops they were given rather than from something picked up as they travelled about London. Even so Andrewes could not support Dochez's claim that in New York they had grown the cold virus on a special type of tissue culture. Dochez was very supportive, even to the point of bringing some of his material over from New York. But even this failed to cause colds in the Bart's students.

It was an interesting start but, evidently, insufficient to justify further expenditure at that time. The MRC decided to terminate the project in 1932. When it emerged that the work on colds had been wound up there were angry questions in parliament and a *Daily Mail* headline announced 'Search for cold cure abandoned', claiming that the disease was 'costing the country £15m a year'. Andrewes turned his attention to research into influenza viruses, the thirties proceeded to a close, and Europe headed inexorably towards a second world war.

CHAPTER 2

Harvard University and the American Red Cross

Common cold research, in spite of these distractions, was attracting considerable support in Britain, and this was largely due to the attention being given to it by certain groups in the United States. *The Lancet* reported in 1930 that $195\,000 had been given to Johns Hopkins Medical School to create the John J. Abel Fund to support research on the common cold. And we have just seen how the study of colds in New York City impressed young Dr Andrewes and the senior MRC staff in Britain. But another important element was the contribution, in 1940, of Harvard University in Boston, Massachusetts—in a quite different but very practical and immediate way.

Harvard, founded in 1636, is the oldest educational establishment in the United States, with interests that stretch far beyond its shores. These interests include a particular affection for Europe, and the reasons for this go right back to the years immediately following its foundation when, quite possibly, it owed its survival to the generosity of an Englishman, a certain John Harvard. Brought up in England and educated at Cambridge University, Harvard emigrated to America in 1637 and died a year later, leaving the university half his estate. The university then adopted his name as a mark of its gratitude.

This outward-looking attitude was strongly evident in 1915 when, with Europe at war but the USA still neutral, the Harvard Medical School sent out a volunteer surgical unit. This worked with the British army in Paris and provided valuable help. But the action which was to have such a bearing on our studies occurred in September 1939 when, once again, Harvard came to our aid. Within 10 days of war being declared Dr James B. Conant, an outstanding president of the university, called a meeting at which they agreed to send us another medical mission. Little was done about this over the next few months, which happened to be winter time, probably because it was the period of the 'phoney war' in which there was very little fighting. It was the calm before the storm.

Came the spring and the situation changed dramatically. The Nazis invaded Norway and Denmark and, by July, France had fallen. The mood in Boston changed too: it was felt that something practical and active had to be

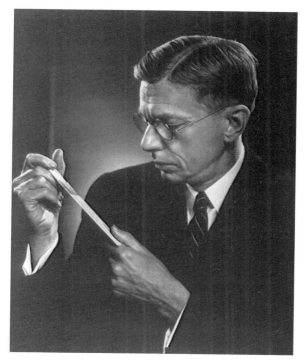

Fig. 2.1 Dr J. Conant, president of Harvard University, Boston, Massachusetts. (From the estate of Karsh of Ottawa.)

done, and quickly. Conant believed there were four areas in which Harvard might help and needed to establish which one the British would prefer. Fortunately he had someone near at hand who could help him find out.

Professor Reginald Linstead of the Harvard Chemistry Department, a British citizen, had been doing research work at the university but was due to return to Britain that July. And so Harvard enlisted him as an envoy and asked him to find out what sort of mission the British Government would like.

An offer gratefully accepted

Linstead was warmly received in London and was told that one of the main concerns was the possibility of epidemics resulting from infectious diseases. Harvard was informed and cables were exchanged. The Ministry of Health was afraid that the movement of large numbers from the cities into the country or the crowding together in air-raid shelters would provoke outbreaks of one sort or another. Their reply was along the following lines: 'we would be very grateful for a mission that would help care for cases of communicable diseases, and with hospital facilities, if possible, because there is a national shortage'.

And so, towards the end of July, there was another meeting in the president's office at Harvard to consider its response. It resulted in the following cable:

> HARVARD READY TO SEND SMALL ADVANCE GROUP OF EXPERT FIELD AND LABORATORY WORKERS INCLUDING GORDON TO LEND TECHNICAL ASSISTANCE LOOKING TOWARD ORGANIZATION OF COMPREHENSIVE UNIT STOP READY TO FINANCE THESE MEN FOR ONE YEAR STOP IF THIS OFFER ACCEPTABLE HOPE TO ENLARGE GROUP LENGTHEN PERIOD OF SERVICE AND EXPAND WORK ALONG LINES OF YOUR CABLEGRAM PROVIDED WE CAN RAISE NECESSARY FUNDS STOP HAVE GIVEN CAREFUL STUDY HOSPITAL PROJECT AND FIND IT INVOLVES CONSIDERABLE DELAY STOP THEREFORE BELIEVE IF NEED URGENT QUICKER FEATURES SHOULD BE INITIATED AT ONCE STOP FUND RAISING FOR ANY PURPOSE INCREASINGLY DIFFICULT AT THIS TIME STOP THEREFORE ASSURANCES FROM BRITISH AUTHORITIES ON TWO POINTS WOULD BE OF GREATEST ASSISTANCE STOP FIRST URGENCY OF NEED OF ENTIRE PROJECT STOP SECOND ACTUAL EXTENT OF CONTRIBUTION BRITISH READY TO MAKE TO SUPPORT OF LARGER PLAN

Two days later a cable from the minister of health, Malcolm MacDonald, gratefully accepted this 'generous offer' and invited Dr John E. Gordon to visit immediately and discuss the questions and develop plans. Gordon was professor of epidemiology in the Harvard School of Public Health.

The Americans thought of the 'comprehensive unit' as being in three parts. One would be a small group of experts in infectious diseases and epidemiology who could study and care for patients who came to them or were identified as needing treatment during investigation of an outbreak. The second would be a fully equipped laboratory for the diagnosis of infections of any sort. And the third would be an equipped and staffed infectious diseases hospital.

Gordon wanted to make personal contact with the British as soon as possible, but travel was not easy. All the ships bound for Britain belonged to belligerent nations and would not welcome citizens of neutral countries on board. Nevertheless they managed to reach London on 13 August 1940, just as the Battle of Britain air raids began. Preparations for sending the unit were immediately begun and they also gave advice on the problems of handling infectious diseases.

Back in the USA money had to be raised, as their cable had indicated. There was a vigorous campaign to contact charities, industry, and private individuals, including some who had served on the previous mission to France. The university staff realised that they would not be able to provide a hospital in the timescale needed, so Conant approached the head of the American Red Cross, knowing that the organisation had the staff and resources to put together an emergency hospital. Fortunately they responded enthusiastically and action quickly followed. It was to be one-third of the whole effort.

The attractions of Harnham Hill

Gordon stayed in England for less than a month, returning to Boston in September, but his time had been well spent. Detailed discussions with our chief medical officer had established what would be required on both sides. He had also been told that there was a suitable site on Harnham Hill, above the village of Harnham on the outskirts of Salisbury. Situated fairly centrally in southern England and reasonably distant from any industrial centres, it was an unlikely target for German bombers. It seemed ideal and, furthermore, it was available. All this and more was reported back to the high-level committee at Harvard that had been set up to drive the project along. Things were beginning to take shape.

Harvard set about recruiting medical and other staff trained in epidemiology and ready to care for patients in the hospital when it opened. Supporting them would be laboratory staff, and so the university also took on the task of gathering the equipment and chemicals which these people would need. And then there was the question of finding a chief physician for the hospital—a key appointment.

Paul Beeson recalls that in September 1940 he was serving as chief resident physician at the Peter Bent Brigham Hospital in Boston, the final stage of his clinical training in the teaching hospitals of the city, when he was approached by the dean of the medical school and asked whether he was willing to take on this wartime appointment in England. He jumped at the chance and, by late December, having been released from his existing duties, he and Gordon were on their way. An American steamer took them to Lisbon where they were picked up by RAF seaplane and flown to Poole on the south coast of England, conveniently near to Salisbury. After inspecting the site on Harnham Hill they travelled on to London to set up their interim headquarters.

For Beeson it was the start of a long and distinguished career in medicine. His duties at the hospital continued until the Americans entered the war in 1941 and their military took over the project. Once this happened he was free to take on the associate professorship which awaited him at Emory University in Atlanta, Georgia, a post that had been held open for him while he fulfilled these wartime duties. Accompanying him on his return to the States was the wife he had met and courted in the grounds of the Harvard hospital. He was later to return to Britain, where he was appointed Nuffield professor of medicine at Oxford University and received an honorary knighthood for his services.

Before he left the US Gordon recruited two experts in public health, John A. Degen Jr and Dean S. Fleming. And for the head of the laboratory research team he selected a Briton who had settled in Pennsylvania, Dr Tom MacNair Scott. Scott, a visiting researcher in paediatrics at Harvard, had made a reputation for himself in pathology and virology, and was willing to volunteer. The American Red Cross, meanwhile, was already in touch with a number of suitable people. Amongst them was Charles (Charlie) Carr who had worked for them in Spain, during the civil war, and elsewhere as an administrator. But they needed many more. Advertisements were placed in the nursing press for trained nursing staff, bringing responses from all over the country. Gertrude Madley, who was born in Britain, was chosen for the post of chief nurse. She had been a founder member of the Royal College of Nursing before she left for the USA.

Once the key positions had been filled it was then a question of deciding what buildings and equipment would be needed on the other side of the Atlantic. Gertrude recalled being provided with an office in Washington and

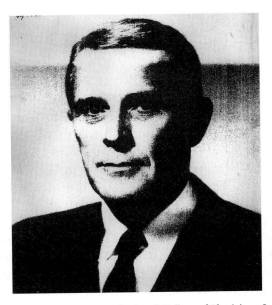

Fig. 2.2 Dr Paul Beeson. (From the Royal College of Physicians, London.)

a pile of catalogues. She was instructed to list and order absolutely everything that the complete hospital would need when they arrived. Meetings were held with medical staff to agree on the various components, the most important criterion being that each item must be available off-the-shelf. Time was short and immediate delivery was essential.

The main structures were obtained from companies that supplied standardised huts, used typically by building, mining, and lumber companies as temporary offices, dormitories, or stores. The hospital had been planned as a series of interconnected huts, each 120 feet long. They were dispersed to reduce the risk of cross infection and of damage from enemy attack. The interiors were to be divided with standard panels and doors to form wards, offices, laboratories, staff quarters, and a recreational area—an early example of a system-built hospital. The plan was to send the materials by ship and assemble them on site.

Gertrude Madley obtained the furnishings, or most of them, in record time. Pine bedroom furniture and domestic units were selected from mail-order catalogues. A complete range of linen, medical supplies, and instruments was also assembled. But it was simply not possible to get all the hospital items in time. Even so there was still too much to go in one ship. The load had to be split between a number of them, with consequences that were both tragic and farcical.

Conant's fact-finding mission

In March 1941 Conant made the hazardous journey to England, embarking on a punishing round of visits to all those with an interest in the project, including the prime minister and university top brass. Later in the month he travelled down to Salisbury, staying at the White Hart Hotel. Although suffering from an unpleasant throat infection at the time, he rallied and found the energy to visit the site and give it his approval. His verdict was 'grand…on a site just on the edge of the town, which looked crowded but peaceful…only seven bombs through all the months'. This statement will give some idea of the level of bombardment elsewhere, particularly in nearby Southampton.

He received a letter of warm appreciation from Sir Wilson Jameson, Britain's chief medical officer, in which he said, 'the inclusion in the Harvard Unit of an epidemiological medical team assisted by trained public health nurses gave me the greatest possible satisfaction…the epidemiological team will be used as though they were members of the staff of the Ministry of Health in whatever part of the country disease has to be investigated and brought under control.'

Conant returned to America on 10 April. Fresh in his mind was the memory of a meeting he had with Winston Churchill in the cabinet room. Amongst the subjects they discussed was the looming disaster in Greece—just one more tragic episode in a war that was not going well. Churchill was clearly disturbed by events as he expressed the dismay felt by people throughout the country: 'Here we are, standing alone. What is going to happen?' It was clearly a plea for help and one of many incidents that made Conant determined that he would speak bluntly to his isolationist friends back home. Their theme was that Britain should be urged to come to terms with Hitler. His reply was that, to anyone who had been in England, such an idea was utterly fantastic. And, he pointed out, 'Though they were subject to a continuous threat of air raids and many suffered directly from night bombing, there was no thought of compromise…no British Government could come to power which was committed to making peace with Hitler.'

Moving to England

Some cynics branded the whole scheme as a bit of a jaunt and the volunteers as self-indulgent, but those who went viewed it differently. Most of them were quite young and not averse to a bit of adventure, but they also saw it as an opportunity to help a people in difficulty and to do something worthwhile with the professional skills they had acquired. And they were quite prepared to swim against the tide of isolationism which was running strongly amongst some groups in the USA.

One of those who came, Martha Reiner, had just finished her training when a friend showed her the Red Cross advertisement in a nursing journal. She thought it would be a task worth doing, now she was qualified, and an opportunity to experience something different. She went ahead and volunteered but remembered feeling increasingly apprehensive as she sat in New York in the summer of 1941 waiting for instructions to leave. All she could do was to stay on in the hotel with her new Red Cross uniform and the very limited amount of personal belongings they were allowed, wondering what was going to happen. Finally their instructions came and with some 14 other nurses and a small party of marines she boarded a Dutch cargo ship, the *Maasdam*.

They sailed as part of a large convoy, stretching from one horizon to the other. Protecting them was an outer screen of naval vessels, but it was not enough. Within a matter of days they were attacked by U-boats and the *Maasdam* was hit. Ordered to abandon ship they donned life jackets and took to the lifeboats. Each was allowed to take only a handbag. Fortunately the weather was mild and they were soon picked up by a Swedish freighter. This took them to Iceland where they were looked after in a nurses' home.

Other nurses in the convoy were less fortunate. They also were torpedoed and five of them together with the house-mother were lost, the remainder spending 19 days at sea in an open boat before they were rescued. Some of them were so badly affected by the experience that they had to be invalided out of the project and returned to the USA.

Some weeks passed before the American volunteers finally made it to England. A British troopship picked up the stranded nurses in Iceland and brought them to Glasgow, where they were greeted by Paul Beeson. In view of their ordeal he had decided that, as chief physician of the hospital, the least he could do was to escort them down to London. Beeson could sympathise with their plight for he, too, had been experiencing the war in a manner that was a little too close for comfort. The London building in which he and Gordon were staying was hit by a bomb. They were there at the time and were blown across the room and cut by flying glass. It was a lucky escape.

The dangers of the Atlantic crossing affected not just personnel but also caused a delay in construction of the hospital. As mentioned earlier, the volume of materials being sent over by the American Red Cross was such that several ships were needed to accommodate them. Amongst these were the prefabricated sections for building the hospital, together with the nuts and bolts necessary for screwing them together. Unfortunately the nuts were put in one ship and the bolts in another, and one of the ships was sunk. History does not record which was lost but one was no good without the other, and so the various panels and beams could not be linked. Nor was it possible to obtain local alternatives. Quite apart from the difficulty of obtaining any engineering products from manufacturers stretched to breaking point to meet the demands of the war effort, screws and bolts were manufactured to different thread standards in the US and Britain. There was nothing for it but to await replacements from America.

England was a very different place

After the nurses reached Britain they had to wait until they could move into the Harvard Hospital, as it later became known. Any frustration or disappointment they felt was tempered by the warm welcome given to them by their opposite numbers and by the public. Fresh uniforms were produced in London to provide an exact match for the ones they had lost at sea. And they were then placed in various hospitals to help look after patients. One of these was St Bartholomew's which had been evacuated to the northern outskirts of London.

England must have seemed very different to the USA. Clothes, houses, food, and customs all had their distinctive British characteristics and, of course, there were wartime restrictions such as food rationing, blackout, travel difficulties, and the ever-present fear of air raids. The British, for their part, found young American men and women interesting too. They had some idea of what to expect from books and the cinema, but to meet real Americans and see their clothes and hear their voices was a genuine novelty. Visitors from the USA were then rare compared with the decades after the war. Mixed with this interest was a strong feeling of gratitude. Many people felt isolated and beleaguered, and these lively young Americans were appreciated for volunteering to come and help.

The delay in construction of the hospital was not a long one and by June the first huts had been completed and fitted out as laboratories. Their task was to carry out diagnostic tests on material sent in by field teams who, since the beginning of the year, had been travelling round the country investigating outbreaks such as paratyphoid and other intestinal infections. Hospital equipment quickly followed and was unpacked and put in place. By the end of summer the large piles of timber that had lain under tarpaulin covers on

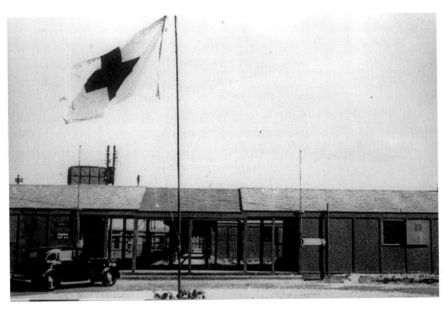

Fig. 2.3 The American Red Cross/Harvard Hospital. (From the collection of Lois Simon.) The area in the foreground was known as Times Square, a name it retained throughout the lifetime of the Common Cold Unit.

that windy hilltop had become 22 fully equipped buildings, including a 125-bed hospital—a great tribute to the American team and the British who prepared the site and did much of the erection. In September 1941 the American Red Cross–Harvard Hospital was opened and the three-part project was in place. The hospital could now receive patients.

The major epidemics that the ministry had feared did not materialise; instead, a trickle of civilian and military cases began to arrive. Some were due to medical activity. For example a British medical officer, Dr (later Sir) Charles Stuart-Harris, was doing research up on Salisbury Plain to develop a vaccine against typhus and became infected with the organism. He was taken to Harvard for expert care. His wife remembered making a fire of his clothes in the garden with the help of Paul Beeson, an example of just how little was

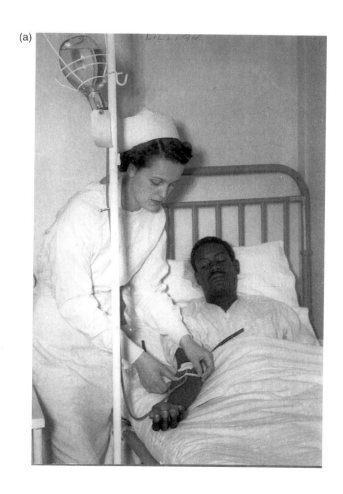
(a)

(b)

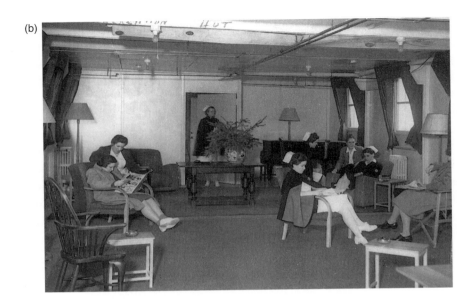

(c)

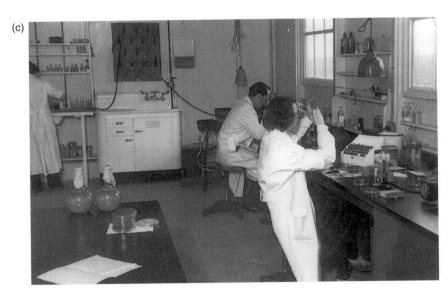

Fig. 2.4 The American staff settle in. (a) A patient receives the special care of an American nurse. (b) Staff relax in the recreation hut. (c) The hospital laboratory, which changed little over many decades. (From the collection of Lois Simon.)

known about how it might be transmitted. All mention of the incident was suppressed, which reflects how anxious the Allies were to avoid giving German Intelligence any idea of where an offensive was being planned. All the same the contribution of the Harvard team was much appreciated in high places; Dr Gordon was recognised as a liaison officer with the Ministry of Health; and the chief medical officer expressed his thanks.

Life and work in the Harvard Hospital

Field investigators from the unit continued doing valuable work around the country and were able to solve a number of problems associated with infectious diseases. Paul Beeson investigated an unpleasant type of poisoning in the north of England which turned out to be due to cysticercosis—a disease that was not well known in Britain. It is caused by a worm that lives in the intestines of pigs and then spends another part of its lifecycle as a small cyst in muscle. When undercooked meat is eaten, the cyst opens and becomes a larva and then a worm once more. Such meat used to be known as measly pork. Solving this particular mystery took some skilful medical work, helped by the fact that Beeson soon realised the condition was something he had seen back in Boston. It all stemmed from contaminated garbage. He discovered that, in Britain, rats were picking up the infection and passing it on to pigs; the resultant measly pork was processed, turned into sausages, and then eaten.

Another team, consisting of a clinician, two bacteriologists, and several nurses went to Bristol to discover the source of an outbreak of paratyphoid fever. Their detective work revealed that it came from eating a wartime substitute for whipped cream that was being produced without adequate hygienic precautions. The rules had to be tightened up.

Unusual infectious diseases were of special interest to the Harvard Hospital, and one particular series of outbreaks intrigued it greatly. This concerned an illness known as cervical myalgia (pain in the muscles of the neck), which seemed to be infectious. So when an outbreak occurred amongst its own staff the unit mobilised all its resources, trying all the bacteriological and virological tests it had available. It even attempted to reproduce the disease by infecting volunteers and thus proving that it was due to an infection. But to no avail—it could not identify any virus or other agent.

Tom MacNair-Scott says that volunteers were recruited in a very informal way and could not be put into isolation but were given blood and swab material. Apparently a few of them showed signs of illness but it was not certain that the disease had been transmitted. Years later interesting viruses that tended to attack muscle were discovered in the USA, in a small town in upper New York State called Coxsackie, and this name was given to the viruses. Later it was found they belong to the enterovirus family and, looking back, I wonder whether they had been the cause of the little outbreak. Although it was not clear what the volunteer experiments meant scientifically, the results of the study were published in the *Journal of the Royal Society of Medicine*. It was the first report featuring the inoculation of volunteers on the top of Harnham Hill.

Another investigation concerned an outbreak of hepatitis (infectious jaundice) amongst a group of British soldiers. Serum from an individual recovered from mumps had been given to them as a protection from the disease. It was clear that hepatitis viruses, which were not well understood at the time, must have been in the serum, as well as the antibody against mumps. The experience was useful when numerous cases of hepatitis occurred in GIs crossing the Atlantic. They had been given a yellow fever vaccine that had been stabilised by the addition of human serum. The hepatitis virus must have been added at the same time.

The US Army takes over

Events began to move fast. In December 1941 the Japanese attacked Pearl Harbor and the USA entered the war. In the spring of 1942 it was decided that the unit would be taken over by the US Army. Many members of the staff wanted to be more involved in the war effort and were immediately commissioned into the army, some of them moving to a nearby, wartime, hutted hospital at Odstock. Some 50 years later, much expanded and modernised, this would become Salisbury's main hospital.

Officially the unit had the title US 5th but because of its origins was usually known as Harvard Hospital. In July it became Medical Laboratory A and later the First General Medical under the well known pathologist Dr (Lieutenant-Colonel) Ralph Muckenfuss. Very quickly it became immersed in a huge volume of work: examining and documenting large numbers of postmortem and surgical specimens; conducting tests in clinical pathology, parasitology, and toxicology as a reference laboratory for many of the smaller hospitals in the European theatre of operations; preparing reagents to send to these hospitals; and running training courses for their staff.

But the laboratory probably contributed most by becoming the main blood transfusion centre for the US Army in Europe. Like the British Army, it had decided that once the invasion of Europe began it must be ready to supply fresh blood in large amounts to treat the wounded. Training those responsible for collecting this became a matter of urgency. John Wallace from the British side (who later became a medical superintendent of the CCU) and his American counterpart set up a training school in Bristol where they ran courses for medical staff.

The war provided exceptional opportunities to hear about the latest research from a broad range of specialists in the field. Wallace recalled travelling down from Hammersmith Hospital, where he had been doing research on blood circulation, to attend a conference at Odstock on blood transfusion. During its course he was able to hear his own chief, Dr (later Sir) John McMichael, speak on the importance of blood replacement and the problems of hepatitis in transfused patients, and then to listen to the views of American experts on the subject. It was a depth of experience he would not have been exposed to under normal circumstances.

Additional facilities were prepared for testing and processing blood. A large cold-storage plant was built, and dispersed around the site was a fleet of vans ready to transport blood to wherever it was needed. Although it was thought originally that blood could be flown in from the US, it was soon realised this would be impractical and that much of it would have to be collected in Britain from non-combatant troops and others.

British and American troops were undergoing training at the time. But once battle commenced in earnest a huge demand for blood transfusion services was expected. The unit made sure it was ready by rehearsing the necessary sequence of operations as a 'dry-run'. Unfortunately these activities were observed and reported by an American journalist who helpfully pointed out that when the invasion was imminent it would be repeated as a wet-run. After that, dry-runs had to be made quite frequently so that any observers would become used to them. Otherwise a sudden, large movement of vans might have warned the enemy that the D-day invasion was about to take place.

After the Normandy landings the Harvard medical and other staff moved on to France, Germany, North Africa, and elsewhere. The laboratories were not so mobile but eventually they were deemed to be too far from the front to do a good job and were moved across to France and eventually to Paris.

Another group attached to the unit were members of the Friends Ambulance Unit (FAU), who did valuable work during the war. Although trained to assist in operating theatres, these skills were not needed during the early stages and, while at Salisbury, they took on the task of assembling and painting hospital equipment. However, their conscientious objections to fighting did not endear them to the US military, as was demonstrated on one occasion when General Eisenhower visited the laboratory. One of the FAU group was detailed to serve tea for the party but, as he reached the door of the room, he was turned back and told he could not enter. Someone else was asked to take it in. The incident, I suppose, was typical of the strong feelings that were aroused in wartime.

The FAU was committed to finding something helpful to do whatever the situation and, prior to the invasion of Normandy, it spent one summer helping a local farmer bring in the harvest. But its refusal to take up arms did not prevent it entering areas of conflict; and when the second front was opened it moved onto the Continent to provide shelter and food for the crowds of refugees who had lost their homes or been driven from their towns and villages by the fighting.

Meanwhile, research on the common cold was effectively abandoned for the duration of hostilities. This was total war involving not only the services but the whole civilian population. Survival, let alone victory, depended on producing food and munitions, coping with bombing and rationing, and maintaining essential services. The health of the nation was important but resources were limited and the problems of the common cold had to be tackled in other ways. The Ministry of Health chose persuasion as its method and ran a number of very good advertising campaigns. One of the best known of these featured excellent colour lithograph cartoons by Bateman and the caption 'Coughs and sneezes spread diseases. Trap the germs by using your handkerchief.'

The big fear was that people, crowded on buses, trains, and in air-raid shelters, would help to spread infectious diseases. And they recognised that even mild infections like colds might be important, interfering with production and possibly leading to more severe illnesses like pneumonia. People had to work and live close to each other but, in the absence of vaccines or other forms of medicine, it was hoped that sensible personal hygiene would cut down the spread of germs.

A red herring

Publicity must surely have helped in this respect—though publicity can be a two-edged sword. There was one item of news towards the end of October 1943 that the MRC could well have done without. But this was still a democracy with a relatively free press and no one censored a report in the *Sunday Express* that seemed to offer something much more effective than using a handkerchief. It claimed that a British scientist had found an 'entirely new remedy' for colds. He had been working in his laboratory, on a novel substance obtained from a mould, when he developed a cold. So he inhaled some of the substance and found that it 'worked with magical speed'. It was exciting

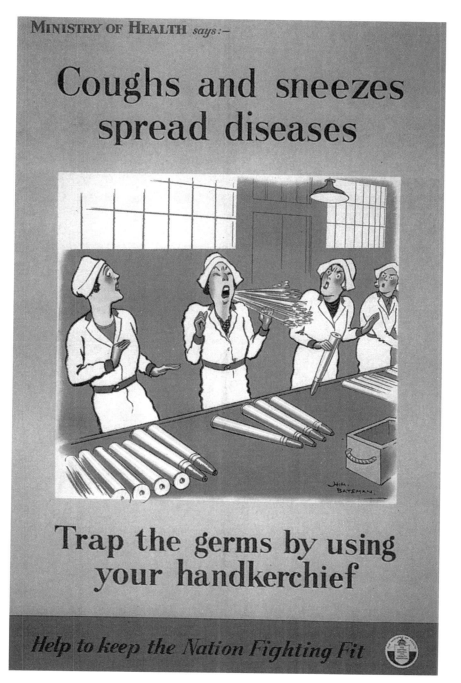

Fig. 2.5 Famous wartime cartoon advertisement from the series by H. M. Bateman.

stuff and, not surprisingly, created quite a stir. The wonder cure was known as patulin and it proved to be a major distraction for all concerned.

The report was a garbled version of a paper by a Professor H. Raistrick of the London School of Hygiene and Tropical Medicine, which he was about to publish in *The Lancet*, the respected medical weekly. There was an immediate and widespread response. Typical was a letter from a representative of the Transport Department of the County Borough of Rotherham in Yorkshire to the MRC, to say that there was a lot of absenteeism in the department, much of it caused by colds. He had read that the MRC had a 'new specific for the cure of common colds' and could it please send him a supply. The Raistrick paper had not yet even been published and the MRC knew little of its content. It certainly had nothing remotely like a cure.

There was a danger that things could get out of hand and the MRC responded with commendable speed, quickly appointing an ad hoc Patulin Clinical Trials Committee on 15 November. The paper was due to be published on 20 November. There were some distinguished members, amongst them Professor Harold Himsworth as chairman (later to become MRC secretary), with Philip D'Arcy Hart as committee secretary. Also included were Major Greenwood, an eminent statistician, and Christopher Andrewes, who was now recognised as an expert on colds. They were under pressure from the outset. Indeed, the week after the paper appeared, a question was put down for answer in parliament by the minister of health asking 'if he has any information to convey to the "House" concerning patulin and whether the drug is being tested on a large scale?'

They decided straightaway that there should be a clinical trial of the substance and that it should take place in multiple centres and over several months in the spring. Letters were sent to the medical officers of various industrial organisations asking them to cooperate. The MRC engaged the Therapeutic Research Corporation (a wartime group of leading pharmaceutical companies) to formulate the drug produced by Raistrick's laboratory and a dummy or placebo preparation. It had learned from an earlier report by an MRC Common Cold Therapy Committee (and no doubt Andrewes confirmed this) that in a cold there were no diagnostic changes to be seen in the nose and throat, and so the best way to diagnose a cold was to ask for typical symptoms. This meant that both the patient and the observer might be biased if they knew, or thought they knew, if the drug had been administered or not. They would avoid this by giving everyone a treatment and keeping both patients and observers ignorant of what they had been given.

swine fever, and then found an influenza virus in animals. The war had largely stopped such work in Britain, but elsewhere influenza viruses continued to be studied, particularly in the USA. Viruses could now be grown readily in eggs containing chicken embryos (embryonated eggs) and detected and analysed using agglutination (clumping together) of red cells, called haemagglutination. And a new type of virus, influenza B, had been isolated and named.

The Australian physician, MacFarlane Burnet, an authority on immunology and viral diseases, divided his history of virology into periods according to the methods employed for their growth. And he reckoned that a second period started in 1940 when many workers began to grow viruses in embryonated eggs. They found that a variety of different, disease-producing organisms could be grown if they were inoculated into the right tissues and organs of hens' eggs that had been incubated for different periods. But were these particular organisms viruses or just fussy bacteria? No one was quite sure but this did not stop investigators, cold researchers included, from trying to make use of the process for any new or difficult infections. Burnet was later awarded the Order of Merit and shared the 1960 Nobel Prize for medicine with Peter Medawar, the Brazilian-born, British immunologist.

Andrewes worked alongside MacFarlane Burnet when he was in London in the 1930s, a period which Burnet regarded as particularly important as he noted in his book. Also working with them was the biophysicist William Elford, who had perfected the use of graduated, collodion membrane filters to calculate the size of particles and then determine their physical properties following high-speed separation in an ultracentrifuge. Between them they showed that viruses were of different sizes and different densities, each with specific antibodies that would neutralise them. It followed that identification of a particular antibody would provide a means of identifying the corresponding virus. This contradicted those people who said that viruses would not stimulate an immune response, making it impossible to vaccinate against them. In saying this, incidentally, they were also ignoring the evidence of smallpox, a viral disease, where vaccination had already been used successfully.

Burnet, Elford, and Andrewes formed a small and very select group, which acquired a level of experience shared by few others at the time. Their fundamental research had brought them a deep understanding of viruses and their behaviour. And they were ready to exploit any opportunities that might present themselves. From the 1930s onwards they were pioneer workers on influenza, and it was the residue and descendants of that group who started work on colds in Britain in 1946. In fact when we grew our first rhino-virus—the largest group of cold viruses—in 1960, we determined the size of the particle using a set of filters prepared by a student of Elford.

Andrewes' hobby was natural history and he continued to wonder about the nature of influenza epidemics. It was part of his heritage for, as a young man, he had been aware of the influenza pandemic which struck the world in 1918; and his father, a pathologist at St Bartholomew's Hospital in London, had done research on the epidemic in Britain. It was difficult to be sure but in some cases it seemed that the infection spread from area to area within countries and indeed from country to country. One of its popular names was 'Spanish flu'.

The World Influenza Centre

Andrewes found himself free from the constraints of wartime work by 1946 and was able to plan new projects for his laboratory in the NIMR in London. The following year he joined a group of 45 people at a planning meeting in Copenhagen; this group appointed a subcommittee of nine and Andrewes prepared a memorandum of its agreed ideas for a scheme to monitor influenza on an international basis. This was presented to the fourth session of the Interim Commission of WHO in September 1947. It approved the proposals and the World Influenza Centre was established under Andrewes at the NIMR.

The plan also called for national influenza laboratories to be set up around the world to collect and study viruses resulting from epidemics in their area. Details of these epidemics were to be passed to WHO in Geneva, and typical strains of virus would go to the World Influenza Centre, soon to be complemented by a similar centre in the USA. The results were then to be collated and distributed. New serotypes of influenza viruses were discovered and tracked across the globe, enabling advance warning to be given to public health authorities of any likely epidemics due to the new viruses. WHO laboratories selected those viruses that seemed likely to be responsible for new epidemics in the coming season and provided suitable strains to manufacturers before the viruses even reached their country. This early warning ensured that the appropriate influenza vaccines could be produced in plenty of time.

WHO maintained high and uniform standards of testing throughout the network by preparing all the standard viruses, sera, and other reagents needed by the national laboratories. And they invited these national groups to send their people for training in the World Influenza Centre laboratories. The whole idea was warmly received and by 1953 there were 54 WHO influenza centres in 42 countries—though they were rather unevenly distributed, with 27 in Europe and 11 in North America. The network is still an established international institution.

Of course, much work is done independently, but WHO is still at the heart of the system for recognising, reporting, and responding to the emergence of new serotypes—from the outbreak of Asian influenza in 1957 up to the present day. In fact when the international community became concerned about the possible spread of influenza viruses to man, WHO added a programme to monitor and study influenza in animals. The H5N1 influenza outbreak in chickens which then affected humans in Hong Kong is a more recent example.

'Another crack at the nut'

Influenza and then wartime duties had diverted Andrewes' attentions away from the common cold, and postwar austerity seemed likely to prevent a resumption of any further research on the subject. A lesser man might have decided to forget the whole idea. But Andrewes was not so easily put off—it was just another challenge to be overcome. And he believed very strongly that, as he put it, 'the time is ripe for having another crack at the nut'. There had to be a way.

He was excited by a report on a disease called primary atypical pneumonia (PAP) by an American scientist Monroe Eaton. During the war this had caused a lot of sickness in US servicemen but, fortunately, few deaths. The illness was thought to be due to a virus, so he had tried out a new method of growing viruses from material such as sputum from patients with various diseases. This involved inoculating incubated fertile hens' eggs in various ways. Although some viruses would kill the embryo in the egg he saw nothing of this sort when he examined eggs that had been inoculated with PAP material and then incubated. But when Eaton took tissue from the embryos and inoculated it into cotton rats or other laboratory animals, they developed a mild type of pneumonia. It looked very much as though in this way he had grown the 'virus' successfully, though other methods had failed. Years later it transpired that the 'virus' was actually a diminutive bacterium, a mycoplasma, but that did not detract from the originality and success of his work.

Andrewes now wanted to try out egg culture on the cold virus but realised he would need human volunteers, at least initially, in order to detect virus. It was, in principle, what Eaton had done with cotton rats and what Andrewes himself had done in the early stages of his work on influenza. He had used a hut in a field at Mill Hill where ferrets could be strictly isolated from the outside world and from each other. He could inoculate them, see whether they got sick, and so discover for certain whether material from the lab contained live influenza or not.

A new kind of ferret house

Work on the common cold with human volunteers required the equivalent of the rigorously isolated ferret house in which Andrewes had first studied influenza virus. It would have to be a building in which human volunteers could live comfortably for 10 days, but in strict isolation, for the duration of an experiment. In 1945 he discussed these ideas with his friend Dr W. H. (Bill) Bradley, an official at the Ministry of Health with a special interest in infectious diseases. Bradley knew that, at Salisbury in Wiltshire, there had been a prefabricated infectious disease hospital provided by Harvard University and the American Red Cross. He also knew it was empty, in good general condition, and now belonged to Britain.

Andrewes then took his ideas to the director of the NIMR, Charles Harington who, in his dry way, gave him his support with the words 'Well, you've got courage.' A small conference of eight scientists met at the NIMR on 11 February 1946 to consider a memorandum from Andrewes in which he put forward his ideas, and from this emerged a series of specific proposals on how it might be implemented, what staff would be required, and so on.

Bill Bradley, who was one of the eight, was enthused by the whole idea and left the meeting determined to do something positive about it. He wanted it to be a joint enterprise with his ministry and in a way which made it possible to tackle the problem properly. A few days later he sent a letter to Andrewes outlining his proposals. They were quite detailed and prepared the way for what was to be the most ambitious attack yet undertaken on the problem of the common cold.

These are the main points of the letter:

> I feel very strongly about the clinical and field aspect of these studies and am sure this side of the work should be no less strong than the laboratory side. We know relatively nothing about the clinical epidemiology of the common cold…I think it would be most unfortunate if you put a lot of work in on the laboratory work without at the same time exploiting the more general studies into the natural history of the disease.
>
> With regard to the place for experiments, you already know that I am not very happy about prisoners and service personnel and that I believe that free volunteers are best. There are many potential sources apart from undergraduates and I do not think we should have difficulty in getting volunteers provided they were approached in the right way and with great enthusiasm.

I have had a talk to Sir Wilson Jameson and other people here. The Harvard Hospital, Salisbury, is the best place we can suggest and there is, in fact, no more suitable building in the country. The Hospital is now standing empty apart from resident caretakers who could easily be turned on to do some of the chores necessary to open the place up for our purpose...I have asked that the Ministry of Works hold their hand until the place has been inspected. When Sir Edward Mellanby has discussed this project with you and if he agrees that we should use the Salisbury place, could you and perhaps one or two others join me in a visit there. I am sure when you have seen the place you will appreciate that it is on the whole very suitable. The staffing and housekeeping difficulties are not of any magnitude. Even at the moment it is probable that the huts are still being heated so as to preserve them. They are furnished satisfactorily and could be brought into use rapidly without disturbing anybody. The same could not be said of any isolation blocks in infectious diseases hospitals.

Bradley was just as enthusiastic and impetuous as Andrewes and felt deeply involved. The letter also showed that he had already softened up key people in the ministry to this strange idea. Using the Harvard Hospital would get the scheme going with the minimum of delay and was a most appropriate way to

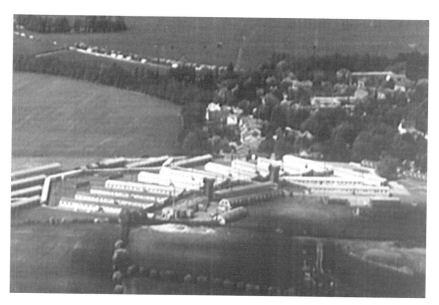

Fig. 3.1 An aerial view of the hospital in its beautiful rural setting, adapted as a volunteer research unit. The six buildings on the left formed the 12 flats for volunteers. The other buildings were adapted to be used for games, laboratories, stores, offices, and staff quarters. (From Aerofilms.)

use the premises. After all, the Americans had given the place to the nation to be used for research.

Andrewes sent the letter on to Sir Edward Mellanby who agreed in April to implement the idea as a joint project. A meeting in early May between the MRC and Ministry of Health clinched the deal; the site was adapted in June and became the Common Cold Research Unit (later shortened to CCU); and the first volunteers' trial began in July 1946. Andrewes was not one to hang about.

A place in the country

Wiltshire now became the focus of activities. Amongst the first to arrive in May was Dr Malcolm Chalmers, a medically qualified member of the NIMR, who was chosen as the first medical superintendent. His immediate task was to design the way in which the new unit would operate. Staff began to take up their appointments. The administrative office required a staff of two—to be recruited locally. A cook, kitchen assistants, and cleaners were also needed. A trained nurse was appointed as the first matron. And, in spite of the shortage of materials and labour, contractors were found to rearrange the walkways connecting the huts.

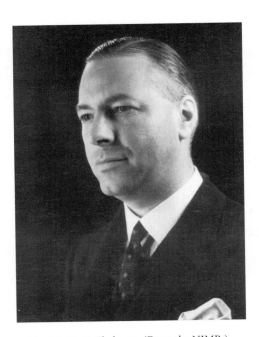

Fig. 3.2 Dr T. Chalmers. (From the NIMR.)

Interior panels were used to make the volunteers' rooms in what had been the staff accommodation, producing two self-contained flats in each of six huts, all with immediate access to the open country. One room in another hut was cleared of animal cages to make way for typists' desks and a telephone. Although possibly intended as a temporary measure, it soon became a permanent feature. It was to remain as the unit office for the next 44 years. The room next door had been used for postmortems but became a laboratory. Huts that had been wards became staff accommodation, laboratories, storerooms, and so on.

In the middle of June a young man recently out of the army arrived. He lived near the NIMR in Hampstead and applied for a job as driver with some general duties. He was struck by the sombre, camouflaged buildings and their contrast with the beautiful countryside around. But, after the desert war in North Africa and grim experiences in Italy, it still seemed wonderful. The man was Keith Thompson (Tom) and he would have been astounded if he could have seen what the future held: he was to spend the rest of his working life on the site. Although starting out as a driver it soon became clear that his abilities qualified him for a much wider range of tasks. Eventually he became executive officer, responsible for the organisation of much day-to-day activity in the unit. He proved to be highly resourceful and a steady, calming influence.

Volunteers were due to arrive in a month and there was much to be done. Flats had to be prepared and hundreds of blackout blinds taken down. Matters were not helped by the limitations of the telephone system. When a call came through someone had to blow a whistle to get the message out across the site. Eventually, and most thankfully, a telephone switchboard and a few extensions were installed.

Perhaps the most important job in those days was to spread the Chalmers attitude that each volunteer was to be regarded as a VIP and made to feel welcome, a conviction that Tom was to pass on to others throughout his life there.

The first volunteer trial

Dropping an unknown fluid into a volunteer's nose and then watching for symptoms over the next five days was the key test in the research programme. Volunteers were to arrive every two weeks, making it possible to conduct a series of systematic experiments and to confirm results previously reported.

By now there were 15 members of staff in residence. It was early July and, whilst there were still things to be done, the main buildings were ready and everyone had learned their part in the Chalmers scheme, more or less. But how would it work out when real volunteers arrived? They would soon find out—the first trial was due to start on 11 July.

Seven students came down from London and were picked up at Salisbury railway station. Their flats were ready to receive them and the telephones were working. The doctor and matron would have to wash their hands in an enamel bowl perched on a stand in the runway outside the door of each flat, but there was a washbasin with piped water for the volunteers inside. They were supposed to have radios but these were difficult to obtain and had not yet arrived. Food rationing, imposed during the war, was still in force and so the volunteers handed in their ration books as soon as they arrived. This ensured that commodities such as butter and meat could be obtained on their behalf. Meals were delivered to each flat door in large thermos containers four times a day. They were told about the strict isolation precautions but, provided they stayed in their pairs and at least 30 feet away from any other person, they were free to play outdoor games—indoor recreation huts were not yet ready—and to go walking or cycling in the country south of Salisbury.

Doctor and matron, wearing surgical gowns and masks, visited them each day at the outset to record their symptoms. This was the initial quarantine

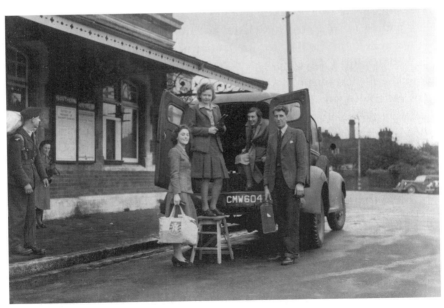

Fig. 3.3 Volunteers arrive at Salisbury railway station to be transported to the unit for the first trial—17 July 1946. Keith (Tom) Thompson is standing on the right. (From Keith R. Thompson.)

period of 3 days, an essential part of every volunteer programme, in which it could be established if any of the volunteers had brought colds with them. If after this period there were no signs of a cold then it could be safely assumed that they had not contracted one prior to their arrival. On the other hand, if anyone exhibited cold symptoms then they could not be used as subjects for the tests and had to be sent home. Inevitably, during the many years of the volunteer programme, some colds showed up in this incubation period, but not on this first occasion. All of them had a clean bill of health and it was possible to move to the next stage of the experiment—dropping fluids into each of their noses to see if colds could be induced.

Everyone was fascinated to see how this historic investigation would proceed. Two scientists and two technicians were in the unit throughout the trial; Andrewes and his technician, Denis Busby, came for the second five days; and Bill Bradley turned up for the final stages. They were hoping that the experiment would provide them with the answers to three important questions. Would the volunteer system prove a success? Would they be able to pass the virus direct from a known sufferer to some of the volunteers and confirm this by detecting it in the noses of the recipients? And would they be able to incubate the same virus in some medium other than the human body and use this to produce a cold?

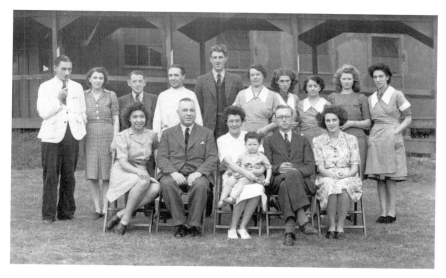

Fig. 3.4 The staff of the CCU, 1946. (From L. Langford.)

The sample fluids they were to use had been produced in the laboratory at the NIMR, Hampstead, and developed from a cold which had affected one of the scientists, Dr Alastair Dudgeon. His nose had been washed out by running a fluid from a pipette into both sides and then tilting his head forward so that the fluid, now mixed with mucus from the nose, could drip into a dish. These washings were passed through a filter to sieve out bacteria. Some of this filtrate was immediately frozen to preserve any virus it contained. The remainder was inoculated into the amniotic cavity of fertile eggs. In those days this was the best way to grow influenza viruses from patients and it was hoped that the method would be equally applicable to cold viruses. A few days later fluid was collected from the eggs and frozen. Dudgeon then sent the samples down to Salisbury.

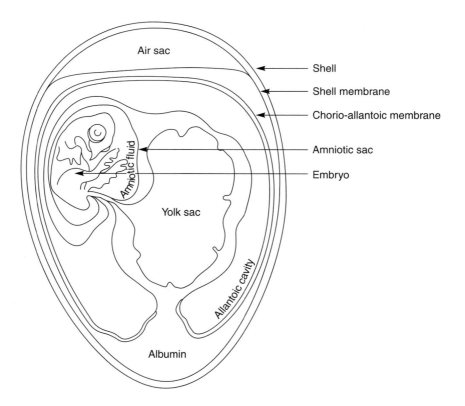

Fig. 3.5 Diagram of an incubated hens egg showing the allantoic and amniotic cavities. A hole was made in the shell and the cavities were inoculated with a fine needle and syringe. The egg was sealed and incubated further to allow the virus to grow for few days. After this it was opened and the fluids sucked out for further testing.

The samples had been placed in small screw-capped bottles, labelled simply A, B, C, or D so that doctors and volunteers were ignorant of what they contained. They were then thawed and a few drops placed in the nostrils of each volunteer. The doctor and nurse visited them each day throughout the trial and noted that two volunteers had developed mild colds. But what had they been given? It was time to interpret the code.

Bottles A and B contained filtered nasal washings, C was the amniotic fluid, and D contained a control fluid—a sterile serum broth. A and B had been given to three volunteers, two of whom had developed colds. C had been given to two volunteers, both of whom had remained well, as had the two volunteers given D. It was a good start.

The scientific staff then assessed what they had learned. The past six months of high pressure work had brought success. They now had a functioning volunteer unit and they could mount a trial. And the result was clear-cut and plausible: they had produced mild colds with a cold virus. The first attempt to grow it in eggs appeared to have failed, but this was not conclusive. The virus might have grown but, by chance, had not produced colds on this occasion. It had only been given to two people and, on average, nasal washings usually produce colds in about one in three volunteers. More people would have to be included in the experiment before they could be certain of the answer. The experiments were cumbersome, it was true, but viruses could now be detected in the noses of people with colds and it was possible to discover some of their properties. And we could test methods of growing them in the laboratory.

So, what was it like?

No one knew at the outset quite how the volunteers would react to the treatment they received or to the conditions in which they were accommodated. In fact the response in those early days was almost entirely positive, and this remained the case throughout the lifetime of the unit. Some experienced an almost sublime sense of peace.

One volunteer from an early trial wrote:

> It was a fine place. I was able to retreat in the monastic sense, once to read, the second time to revise for an impending examination. Everything was gently controlled and, although the Scottish matron was somewhat unnerving and terrifying, the lack of authority, apart from the very few things we were forbidden, was a good relaxation after a heavy term of teaching. And I was given a cold on neither visit.

Another teacher, a woman, came six times in 11 years, always bringing her teddy bear—and, after the first visit, managed to persuade sister to attend to

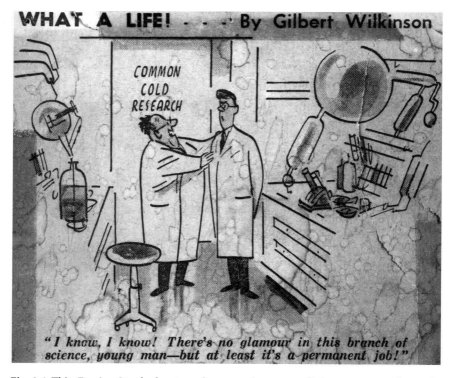

WHAT A LIFE! · · · · By Gilbert Wilkinson

COMMON COLD RESEARCH

"I know, I know! There's no glamour in this branch of science, young man—but at least it's a permanent job!"

Fig. 3.6 This *Evening Standard* cartoon hung on the mess wall for many years (hence its condition) to raise staff morale on bad days!

it as well as its owner. Such harmless make-believe and a number of other pursuits kept her fully occupied:

> Time flew, sewing, reading, going on the occasional walk. It was a complete break from the world, a time to return to the freedom of childhood without its restraints. The yellow trolley (bringing meals) was a highlight of the trials. Pavlov's dogs had nothing on us. We always looked forward with eager anticipation to it coming round. Not that we were ever hungry. Although I recognise the importance of the research, for me personally the social side of the CCU was important. However you matched complete strangers I will never know...I never found myself sharing with anyone I disliked. The buildings certainly gave the impression of a POW camp—but only in looks. The atmosphere was extremely friendly.

Surprisingly, many of the volunteers were quite eager to catch a cold, even to the point of imagining the symptoms. But there were others who, whilst enjoying their stay at the unit, were very keen to avoid any such unpleasantness. Andrewes' eldest son, John, was a student at Cambridge and went as a volunteer to three of the early trials. 'Nobody succeeded in giving me a cold', he said. 'I indulged in a rigorous programme of cold baths each morning in the hope of forestalling this, so whether I actually frustrated my father's plan or not, I do not know.' Such tactics showed something of his father's inventiveness, and this was again demonstrated in thinking up ways of passing the time, particularly in the evenings. He and his flatmate were friendly with a girl attending the trial and, as he explained, 'used to play the most extraordinary games over the telephone, like three-dimensional noughts and crosses and charades.'

Eventually, as the years passed, there evolved a collection of photographs, drawings, poems, etc., put together by the volunteers, which provided a sort of running commentary on life at the unit for the benefit of those who came later. It was a source of much interest and some amusement—particularly with such cartoons as 'Run or your nose will' and a 'Colditz' sketch harping on the prison camp aspect.

After each trial, volunteers were given their travel expenses, which varied between 19s 8d (approximately 98 p) and £1 17s 5d (about £1.87), said their goodbyes, and returned home. They left behind a few suggestions. Typical of these was the following list of wants:

1. mats and cushions in the flats
2. Bovril, Marmite, paste or chocolate-spread to make the jam ration go further
3. a Sunday paper
4. Something to heat milk (noted in the office to be 'not practical')

A breath of fresh air

During these early days the CCU was providing a home to a different, but related, branch of scientific research. During the war there had been problems of infection in air-raid shelters and elsewhere, and so the MRC had formed an Air Hygiene Unit at the NIMR in Mill Hill. It was a small section staffed by two bright young PhD scientists, James Lovelock and Owen Lidwell. But the NIMR was short of space and so Lovelock and Lidwell were persuaded to move down to Salisbury, where there was plenty of room and every likelihood that their work would impinge upon that of the CCU. They were both married with children and so there was the added attraction of good, cheap living accommodation in a pleasant country setting.

They formed an interesting pair: one studious and thoughtful, the product of a fairly privileged upbringing, and the other lively and unconventional, from what would then have been described as a working-class family. Lidwell

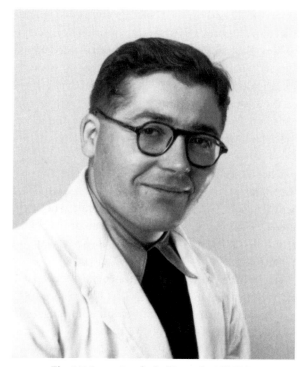

Fig. 3.7 James Lovelock. (From the NIMR.)

was educated at St Paul's School in London and Oxford University. Lovelock's rural background may have been somewhat humbler but he had the advantage of parents with intelligent, inquiring minds: a father interested in nature and a mother who was an avid reader. As a small boy he demonstrated his technical capabilities by making his own radio set from a box of electrical parts, and he learnt about science by reading books from the local library. He went straight from school to a commercial analytical laboratory, but fortunately his exceptional talent was recognised and he was awarded a university scholarship, leading to a PhD degree.

The CCU provided them with a laboratory and workshop and they quickly became part of the scientific and social life of the unit. Lidwell, at the time, was studying the prevention of airborne infection in London schools and was able to continue this while at Salisbury. He also joined in a number of CCU projects. Later he moved to the Central Public Health Laboratories in London but, after retirement, came back to use our facilities while studying the implications of cross-infections during hip replacement operations.

Lovelock proved to be a pleasant and amusing companion, on and off duty—and very resourceful. This was well-illustrated by his contribution towards stress-free fishing, devising an electrical method to bring worms to the surface rather than digging them out. He also produced an instrument for measuring airflow based on a small radioactive source, but discovered that it failed if someone nearby was smoking. He deduced that it must be sensitive to chemicals in the tobacco smoke, and so developed it as an extremely sensitive detector of biologically active substances, such as those that produce cancer and those used in insecticides. Moving to the NIMR he incorporated this idea into the newly developed gas chromatography apparatus, which could separate and identify such molecules.

It was inevitable that a man of such wide-ranging talents would find the MRC organisation a little too restricting but it did give him, particularly at Salisbury, the resources and freedom to launch his remarkable career as an independent scientist. His work on environmental pollution led to his being engaged by NASA to design instruments to be sent to Mars to look for signs of life. And it was this that prompted him to formulate the hypothesis for which he is now famous. He called it Gaia, the idea that our planet is a self-regulating system in which all matter, both living and non-living, forms a single entity which is not only conducive to life on earth but actively maintains it.

The CCU was now clearly in business. Everything was functioning well. Research facilities were basic but adequate. There was no great difficulty in attracting the necessary number of volunteers. And the Harvard Hospital site was proving ideal for the programme of work that was envisaged. The road ahead was clear: they must do more trials and they knew now that they could. But it was to be a very long road.

CHAPTER 4

Uncertain beginnings

The CCU was set up so that the team could find out how to grow the cold virus in the laboratory. But catching and taming a virus is like stalking an animal. It has to be approached with extreme care and in a roundabout way. The initial result of their experiments would be a slightly cloudy fluid in a tube. But that could be anything. They had to be absolutely certain it had a live virus in it that would reliably produce colds. If they could achieve that it would be a major advance in cold research. Meanwhile their experiments with volunteers had to rely upon transfers from known sufferers.

First results were promising. The volunteers were given nasal drops made from the nasal washings of cold sufferers. And both experimenters and 'guinea pigs' were delighted to find that as a result they got colds. Making certain that this was so was not as simple as it might seem. Some volunteers got mildly scratchy throats or other non-specific symptoms, and so it was important to decide what signs and symptoms betokened a real cold. Once these were established to the satisfaction of the experimenters they were checked systematically by using a double-blind, controlled design for every test—where neither experimenter nor volunteer knew what was being dispensed.

But is it a virus?

Something in the washings had produced a cold, that was certain. But it might have been a bacterium, an irritant chemical, or something else. More experiments were needed to show that it had the properties of a virus. One study showed that it could be passed on from one group of volunteers to another, apparently indefinitely. This meant it must be multiplying and therefore some sort of living organism. Collodion membrane filters were then employed as a series of sieves to determine its size. It passed through a filter that held back bacteria but was retained by one with a finer pore size. So it was bigger than a protein molecule and smaller than a bacterium. A virus must be the answer but, too small to see with a light microscope and with electron microscopy still in its infancy, it could not be subjected to any significant examination. It could only be classified as some sort of filter-passing virus, though these laborious experiments suggested it could be a relatively small one. Like other viruses it was found that it could be kept alive for long periods by storing it at low temperatures, particularly at the temperature of dry ice (solid CO_2), about $-65\,°C$. This was useful, practical information.

This was the first time that such basic and systematic studies had been done with volunteers. The results were scanty but clear, and they provoked a great deal of interest when Andrewes reported them in lectures and articles in Britain and the USA. More importantly, it meant that the unit had finished with the preliminaries and was ready to attempt what it had been set up to do: to grow the cold virus in the laboratory.

In 1946 the usual method when growing a new virus was to inoculate it into animals. If they became ill you knew that the virus had grown. This had not been tried with the cold virus but there were anecdotes that suggested it might work. One cat owner said that when he got a cold his pet had snuffles too. And so various animals were inoculated with cold washings. This involved quietening them with anaesthetic and then giving the virus as nasal drops. On awakening they were watched for some days for signs of a cold. Finally tissue from the nose was examined under a microscope for signs of disease. The results were negative. But there were plenty more animals to try.

A tale of two pigs

Some experiments were quite eventful. Amongst the animals acquired were two pigs, a situation which generated some excitement and not a little anticipation. These emotions were aroused, not by any special characteristics of the pigs, but by the fact that, after the experiment, the plan was to use the heads for scientific purposes and eat the rest. Anyone from wartime Britain will know what this prospect meant to a meat-starved population. But the unit was not licensed as an abattoir and the staff were not licensed butchers. The problem was soon solved: a butcher would come from Salisbury and kill the animals. Nice idea, but then the Ministry of Food stepped in and said they must have the carcasses.

Things looked desperate for a time, but help was at hand. Dr Somerville, the medical superintendent, was friendly with the local medical officer of health, and he was persuaded to counter this proposal by threatening to declare the meat unfit for human consumption. Inevitably there was a compromise: the unit was allowed to keep one carcase and the ministry took the other. The pig which stayed at home eventually provided a roast-pork feast to remember. No doubt the man who had made it all possible, the local medical officer, was invited.

Some wild hedgehogs also provided their share of amusement or rather, bemusement. Caught locally, the problem with them was a matter of personal hygiene: they were so full of fleas that they had to be dusted liberally with insecticide before they could be inoculated. Then, as hedgehogs are wont to do, they each rolled up into a ball. Any closer approach now became a little tricky but, as the anaesthetic began to take effect, they relaxed a little. Nevertheless there were still some prickles to contend with before the drops were safely up their noses.

In time the cold virus was dispensed to a considerable menagerie. Amongst those getting the treatment were mice, rats, guinea pigs, cotton rats, rabbits, voles, hamsters, grey squirrels, hedgehogs, ferrets, kittens, pigs, green monkeys, red patas monkeys, capuchin monkeys, baboons, and a sooty mangabey. The common species were tested at the unit, while Andrewes took material to London to test on the more exotic creatures. None of them suffered any discomfort, each animal providing the same response: tissues completely normal and no sign of disease. The truth had to be faced, certain viruses will grow in certain animals, and these are the ones which have been identified in the past. But this was clearly not going to be true for the cold virus—animals, in the main, simply do not catch colds. Our best contender and closest relative, the chimpanzee, was not a practical proposition for the CCU, being expensive to look after and difficult to handle.

Andrewes constantly monitored the work of the unit, travelling down to Salisbury by train each time a volunteer trial was in progress, staying for a couple of days on each occasion, supervising tests, and encouraging those who were carrying out the lab work. This kindly, avuncular man had a genuine concern for those who worked for him, dispensing advice, and infecting everyone with his enthusiasm for cold research. They were like an extended family to him, and he treated them almost as a father would his children. Further evidence of this emerged when he indulged in another great passion of his life—natural history.

He had been a keen naturalist since early boyhood, an interest which had developed, as so often happens, during an illness. Confined to his home for a period, he had passed the time by studying the territorial habits of birds in his garden—clear evidence of his innate instinct for research. Eventually he focused his attention on diptera: two-winged flies. And of course his frequent visits to Harnham Hill provided him with an ideal opportunity to pursue these studies. Each morning, during his stay, there was the familiar sight of this figure in a well-worn sports jacket and carrying a net striding out into the countryside, usually along an ancient track, known as the Roman road, and usually accompanied by one of the young laboratory assistants. He would then spend the next half an hour or so giving his companion an insight into the local flora and fauna.

Can an egg catch a cold?

It was depressing but not surprising that none of the animals caught colds. If they did someone would probably have spotted it before. But by the late 1940s there were some new methods, and research from round the world was showing that, for many viruses, these were convenient and effective. They were based on inoculating incubated, fertile hens' eggs. For example, the viruses of illnesses such as influenza, yellow fever, or mumps would multiply if injected into one or other part of the developing embryo. New-grown virus could be collected from the egg fluids. In fact, as we have seen, Andrewes was stimulated to start the unit by reading a report from an American laboratory that the cause of a certain type of pneumonia had just been shown to multiply in eggs.

American journals announced that scientists there had inoculated cold virus into eggs and detected it in the fluids collected some days later. But Andrewes was a stern critic of laboratory standards and methods of detecting the cold virus by inoculating volunteers, and he was not convinced by these reports. But he was impressed by a recent paper from a Dr Tom Ward in the *American Journal of Tropical Medicine and Hygiene*. Ward wrote that not only had he grown the virus in eggs and produced colds, but that he had detected it in the eggs by using the new radioisotope-based biochemical techniques to show changes in the metabolism of the eggs. This method suggested a real breakthrough. It must be tried at the unit.

Someone with experience of bacteriology was needed for the work and the unit's only bacteriologist had recently moved to Birmingham. Andrewes was looking for a replacement but such people were not easy to find; in those days they were mainly medical graduates. Professor Alan Downie of Liverpool University was consulted, and he suggested a certain James Porterfield who had just finished an MD project studying bacterial endocarditis, an infection of the lining of the heart usually due to a common bacterium, the green streptococcus. Although coming from a family of doctors Porterfield had decided not to go into general practice, planning to become a cardiologist instead. Downie thought that more experience of research would be good for his training.

Porterfield came from a village near Widnes on Merseyside. As a child he was good at mathematics but the vigorous walks that were encouraged while he was at boarding school stimulated an interest in natural history. This led

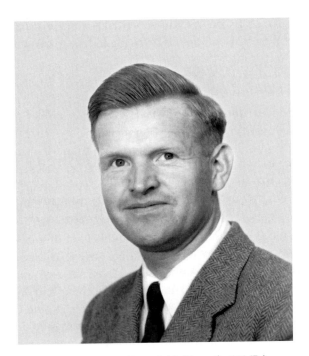

Fig. 4.1 Dr James Porterfield. (From the NIMR.)

him to enter the Medical School in Liverpool, and it proved to be a formative period in his life. This was wartime and, as with so many others, it gave his education an unexpected, and possibly unwelcome, broadening through seeing its effects at close range. Apart from being endangered by the heavy bombing which the city suffered, the students were called on for help when train-loads of wounded arrived from the battlefront in France.

Bacteriology was Porterfield's chosen subject, but while at Liverpool he was also exposed to some of the new ideas concerning viruses. This came about because his professor of bacteriology, Downie, also happened to be a pioneering virologist, and he was in the habit of holding lively discussions on the subject in his department. Porterfield went along to these and was hooked.

Going to work on an egg

The CCU appointment, when it came, followed the casual process with which I was to become familiar. Invited to visit the NIMR at Hampstead, Porterfield was interviewed by Andrewes and the director, Sir Charles Harington. No formal offer was made but he was given a flask of virus to take down to Salisbury

and makes no mention of the interesting background to its beginning: the US onslaught on the poliovirus.

Research into the causes of this disease was given huge impetus through the influence of President Roosevelt, who was severely paralysed following an attack of poliomyelitis in his youth. Initially he helped affected youngsters by organising summer camps, but the epidemics continued and appeared to be getting worse. The general public was distressed and there was an outcry for more practical help, such as respirators (iron lungs), splints, and rehabilitation.

The National Foundation for Infantile Paralysis sprang into action with its famous fund-raising campaign, the 'March of Dimes', which began in 1938. Millions of dollars were collected both to help patients and to support and push forward research on the virus that caused the condition. Outstanding virologists were recruited as advisers and collaborators, and in 1948 it supported an international congress to review the disease. The foundation also funded a very cumbersome animal experiment which demonstrated that the virus existed in three serotypes. Thus it realised that vaccination would be the best way to deal with the mounting epidemics of the disease and determined to support methods to produce virus for vaccine.

Meanwhile there were more promising, indeed exciting, reports just emerging. The source was Dr John Enders, a mature scientist and a man of old-world courtesy and charm, who worked with a few young colleagues in a small laboratory in aged buildings at Harvard Medical School in Boston. They were trying to grow viruses that cause childhood infections and were using cultures of human tissue fragments in flasks or attached to the walls of test tubes with plasma clots. To their surprise they found that poliovirus, which was said not to grow in tissue culture, grew and damaged the cells so that the degeneration could be seen with an ordinary light microscope.

Andrewes saw that this could be the way to grow the cold virus and looked about for new recruits who could set up this type of work at Salisbury. He needed someone who understood cells and how to grow them and someone else with an interest in research on viruses. For the first role he found two people. One was Annette Gompels, a South African spending some time in England. The other, Donna Chaproniere, was British and had studied cell biology, but was less interested in viruses. He recruited his third assistant from South America.

The man from Rio

Helio Pereira grew up in Brazil, qualified in medicine there, and became interested in virus infections. Research in this field was what intrigued him but, at the time, there were few opportunities in his own country. And so, after the war, he applied for and won a British Council Scholarship to Britain. It was an eventful trip: he studied viruses in Manchester and fell in love with a fellow student, Peggy Scott. On completing his studies he spent some enjoyable weeks at the NIMR in Andrewes' lab, after which he married Peggy, returned to Rio de Janeiro, and started a family. Jobs in various laboratories followed but he was unable to find an opening for full-time research. Andrewes, however, had not forgotten him. A letter was sent to Pereira offering him a post at the CCU in Salisbury. It was the opportunity he was looking for and he accepted readily.

Years later, Helio Pereira wrote to me and threw further light on how he had been recruited. Chance once again had played its part. Following his training in Britain and return to Rio in 1947, he had resumed working as a clinical pathologist in a government hospital. But he was unable to pursue his interest in virology. He then transferred to the Instituto Oswaldo Cruz where he developed quantitative techniques for the study of some local diseases due to rickettsia,

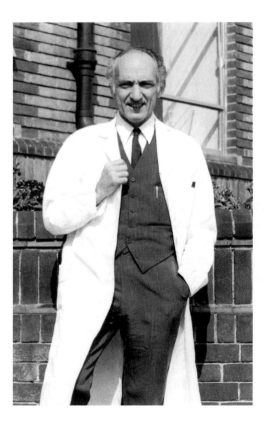
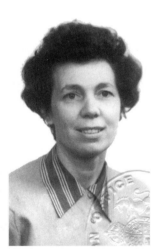

Fig. 4.2 Dr Helio Pereira and (inset) Peggy Pereira. (From the NIMR.)

a small bacterium which causes a number of typhus-like illnesses. In 1950 he was secretary of the Executive Committee for the Fifth International Congress of Microbiology which was taking place in Rio. Andrewes was one of the delegates, and also present was another colleague from England, Sam Cowan.

Andrewes quickly summed up the situation. Pereira's virology skills were being wasted. Soon afterwards Peggy wrote jokingly to Cowan asking him to let her know if he heard of 'any job in virology, somewhere nice in the UK, with board and lodging provided and someone to look after the children so that she also could get a job'. The letter from Andrewes, offering Pereira virology work at the CCU, arrived almost by return of post. They never found out whether Cowan had passed on the message but the job precisely matched her specification in every detail.

The Pereiras sailed from Rio in November 1951 and were met at Southampton docks by a reception party headed by Andrewes. Helio Pereira was most touched by this solicitude. The contrast with the southern hemisphere summer they had just left must have been extreme but caused them no concern—as he pointed out in his letter: 'Living conditions at the Harvard Hospital exceeded our expectations: comfortable accommodation with ample space for ourselves and the children both in and outdoors, more than adequate catering and the friendliest possible neighbours. The staff spared no effort to make us feel at home and to make it easy for me to start work.'

It was the beginning of an illustrious career.

Everything else slotted into place: the children were well looked after and Peggy got her job, first in the clinical laboratory of Salisbury Infirmary and later as head of a newly opened Public Health Laboratory Service in Salisbury.

Pereira initially underwent training at the Strangeways Laboratory in Cambridge prior to establishing tissue culture techniques in Salisbury, and then began the attempt to propagate the cold virus in tissue cultures. The difficulties which attended this project were considerable but, as he made clear, did not detract from his enjoyment of the work:

> My slight fear that I would be working in relative isolation, out of the mainstream, proved unfounded. Andrewes' frequent presence in Salisbury and my regular fortnightly visits to NIMR Mill Hill kept me in touch with what was going on and made it easy for me to make friends and to benefit from their help. Besides, the CCU was a favourite port of call for visitors from within the UK and from other countries. For a beginner like me it was a great thrill to have direct contact with so many famous virologists who came from all over the world. The unit had ideal conditions to accommodate visitors and to provide rewards of both scientific and touristic interest. It was a great privilege for me to join one of the most prestigious and productive virus research groups in the UK, not to say the world.

Pereira took British citizenship in 1957 and, on leaving the CCU, was offered a permanent job at the NIMR, where he became director of the World Influenza Centre (1961–67) and head of the Division of Virology (1964–73). His work was highly regarded throughout the world and led to him being elected a Fellow of the Royal Society.

Donna had a cold

Pereira and his family settled into a flat in one of the huts on the austere site. It was a far cry from the warmth and exoticism of Rio. But he was made welcome, and he had work to do. Pereira was a family man, fond of company but with a quiet and thoughtful disposition. He began, with Donna Chaproniere, setting up the new techniques. He was a particularly skilled and careful experimenter, and she looked upon him as an excellent teacher and guide. They made a patient and competent team.

In those days it was not possible simply to order the materials you needed from a catalogue. Budget restrictions in those post-war years, shortages and, in some cases, the complete absence of many products, meant that you had to use your own initiative. Equipment and reagents had somehow to be produced from whatever was available. The Enders team had described in detail the apparently simple procedures that they used. For example, they cleaned the glassware carefully with a brush and soap flakes. And they used a 'witches' brew' of natural materials to give the cells the nutrients they needed. A source of these in Salisbury was urgently needed.

The answer was to make friends at the local slaughterhouse. They would then be told if a cow was found to be pregnant. When this happened someone hurried into town to collect the amniotic fluid surrounding the calf so it could be checked and stored in the lab to feed the cells. Horse serum, another important component, could be bought, but it had to be checked because some batches were poisonous for cell cultures. The only ingredients they could use off the shelf were the antibiotics they added in small amounts to control bacteria. Finally, they needed an apparatus in which to roll their test-tube cultures. This was necessary because it was known that in order for cells to grow well they needed to be regularly and alternately exposed both to the culture medium and to the air. Slowly turning or rocking the cultures achieved this dual exposure. The institute workshops helped them in this, designing and building a small roller apparatus that would fit inside their incubator—actually a warm cupboard.

Almost everything was ready for the crucial experiment. All they needed was a virus, and suddenly they found one readily available: Donna had a cold.

Quite an ordinary cold and not particularly severe, but it was good enough and a chance not to be missed. It was their policy always to collect genuine cold specimens—and she was quite sure hers was genuine. Nose washings were collected and stored away as a number of little samples in the dry ice

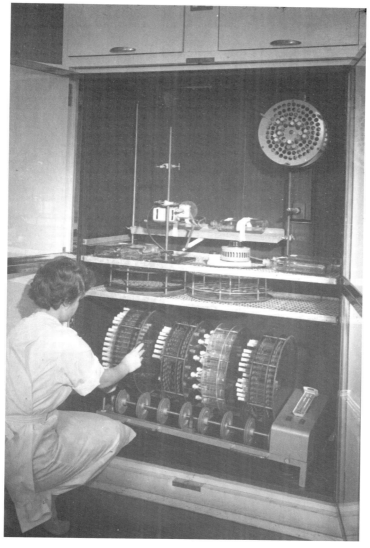

Fig. 4.3 Roller drums in an incubator (warm cupboard) and loaded with test-tube cultures of living cells for growing viruses. (From A. J. Beale.)

freezer. Human lung tissue was used to make as many roller-tube plasma clot cultures as they could. And within a few days they were delighted to see cells growing out of the fragments. So the medium was changed on a few tubes and a sample of Donna's washing was thawed and dropped into them.

The tubes were set to roll in the incubator and every day or two taken out for checking. The cells looked fine and periodically the medium was changed to keep them healthy; but they showed no sign of the degeneration Enders had seen with polio. They knew that viruses might take time to get used to growing in strange cells, so they planned to give them further opportunities to develop. The idea was that, like other viruses, the new virus would gradually change, growing better and better in each set of fresh cells until, in the end, it would kill them; and this would be seen by examining the culture. The laboratory jargon for this was 'adapting' the virus by 'serial passage'. More tubes were taken from the existing batch and inoculated with medium from those given nasal washing, hoping that they would 'adapt' the virus by this 'passage'. But still there was no degeneration. The series was continued until they had made nine passages, by which time they had used up all their cultures. But still there was no degeneration.

They were not prepared to admit defeat. One special, and quite unique, resource remained—the supply of human volunteers.

A stay of execution

Andrewes explained what happened next in a report to the MRC on 8 April 1953.

> Since the beginning, nearly seven years ago, the primary objective has been to find methods for studying the virus apart from the cumbersome volunteer-technique. After $6\frac{1}{2}$ years' failure to achieve this, we were almost prepared, last January, to give up the unequal contest. Even the human cultures of which we were so hopeful, were not yielding encouraging results.
>
> The trial of February 10th–20th, 1953 changed the picture; a fifth subculture of cold virus in human embryo lung gave two colds in six inoculated people. Since then we have had similar results with sixth, eighth and (twice) ninth cultures: on the whole the takes have been nearly as good as with the common cold washings themselves...In the last trial (March 24th—April 2nd) thirteen people received culture medium plus cultivated cells *without* virus: no colds resulted...With things looking so hopeful, this would seem to be a very inopportune time to consider closing down the Unit...If we do not follow up the lead ourselves, our hard-won advantage will be forgotten and another American triumph will probably be acclaimed!

His appeal for support succeeded. The MRC reported the encouraging results in a September press release, at the same time asking for volunteers to come forward to add to the 2496 who had helped the work to that point. This was accompanied by the irresistible offer to pay fares up to a maximum of £3, with three shillings (15 p) a day pocket money. That appeal also succeeded.

Andrewes had enthused the MRC with what he saw as the major developments that would follow this breakthrough: 'an enormous programme of work could be envisaged; it was likely to be as fruitful as the influenza studies of 1933; it would become possible to test for virus by inoculating tissue cultures instead of volunteers'; and so on. This was, as always, a really stimulating phase of a research programme, when scientists let their enthusiasm and imagination take control. Discussions which might normally be confined to the working day spill over into leisure periods. At such times I have seen five minutes over the coffee cups generate enough ideas for five years' work by a laboratory team.

The MRC was, quite rightly, impressed by the unit's persistence, skill, and final success, and agreed to extend support for another three years. It was a tremendous boost. Now all they had to do was to repeat the Donna Chaproniere (DC) experiment and make careful studies of the cultures so they could begin to detect the growth of the virus without inoculating volunteers.

More embryo lung tissue was obtained, cultures were set up and the cells grew well. Then they were inoculated and harvested as before. There were no changes to be seen in the cells, which was not surprising, but when in due course the medium was inoculated into volunteers there were no colds either. It was a clear negative result—the virus was not growing. They were at a loss to know the reason but were determined to continue. The experiment was repeated over the next three years, whenever materials were available, but without success.

The failure was particularly galling because every few months evidence was published showing that tissue culture methods were good for growing new viruses. But having climbed to the top of the hill and seen the promised land it seemed that they had quickly descended to a valley as dark and frustrating as it had been before they grew the DC virus.

A lack of culture

Much of this successful work on growing new viruses in tissue culture was being done in the USA. For example, at the National Institutes of Health they cultured tonsil tissues taken from children at operation. Long narrow cells grew out at first, as expected, but then they shrank into little balls and clustered together like bunches of grapes—an effect known as 'rounding up'.

They were able to show that this rounding up was due to a virus by putting culture medium into cultures of healthy cells, which then degenerated in the same characteristic way. Similar viruses were being found by inoculating material from throat swabs of people with feverish sore throats and similar conditions. They were called APC (adenoidal–pharyngeal–conjunctival) viruses—easy for Americans to remember because these were the initials of a popular tablet for colds and sore throats, containing aspirin, phenacetin, and codeine.

At Salisbury they cultured tonsils collected during operations in the local hospital and found similar viruses growing out. But were they the elusive common cold virus? One way to answer this question was to give nose drops containing the virus to a few volunteers. Some became infected and the virus could be detected in their throats, and some of these developed respiratory symptoms. The clinical observer (the medical superintendent) noted them carefully. The main symptom was sore throat and some fever too, but this was different from the runny nose without fever that affected volunteers given DC or 'pedigree' cold strains. So they concluded that this was one of the group of 'new' viruses and that it certainly caused illness. But it was not the true cold virus as found in typical cases of common cold. In any case they could not culture APC viruses from washings that caused typical colds.

Helio Pereira was fascinated by the organism and began to study its properties in the laboratory. One of his projects was to work on methods of detecting the antigens of the particle and the antibodies produced against them. It was a real relief from the frustrations of DC experiments. And he determined that when he had done his best in hunting for the cold virus he would like to study the strange properties and structure of these 'adenoviruses' as they came to be called. He particularly liked to work on one known as the type 5 virus, which he had first grown at Salisbury, and laughingly referred to himself then as an 'adenovirologist type 5'. After leaving the CCU he continued his research into these viruses.

While still at the unit he and Donna tried to work out general principles of how viruses grew in tissue cultures using chicken viruses and chicken cells. John Hotchin, a new member of staff who had spent time in leading virology labs in the USA, worked on methods of doing the new plaque assays and biochemical tests for infection. But none of this solved the problem of how to get the DC virus to grow.

It seemed the CCU had run into a brick wall. A change of direction was needed. Both Pereira and Donna Chaproniere had developed interests in other aspects of virus research and it seemed right that they should have the opportunity to pursue these. But that meant inviting someone else to take up the challenge if cold research in Britain was not to disappear by default.

International recognition

The unit was now famous internationally and recognised to be unique. Andrewes had given unusual and stimulating lectures in many places. His warm invitations and the striking paper in *The Lancet* about the DC virus ensured that there was a steady stream of visitors, including distinguished individuals. Macfarlane Burnet was amongst them. Another was Harry Eagle.

Eagle was a cancer research worker from the USA who had made valuable contributions to techniques for growing cells. These included the use of specially clean glassware and the synthetic Eagle's medium which he had developed. On asking Donna where she obtained the water for her cultures she replied that she purified it from tap water. This came from two water towers which rose up in the middle of the site. Nothing wrong with that, it seemed, except that the occasional dead pigeon had been found in the towers. But the tanks were thoroughly cleaned and the water purified before it was used. Harry Eagle was not impressed and felt that with water like that she would never be able to do tissue cultures well.

All this worthwhile activity did not alter the fact that they had made no progress in culturing the cold virus. Not for the first time it was pointed out that a small laboratory in 'temporary' buildings, already over 10 years old, was not the place to do high-quality biological research. The purpose of the place was to grow the cold virus. The team had worked hard and it was time to let them have a chance to work in the parent lab of the NIMR, now installed in a specially designed building at Mill Hill with a wide range of up-to-date facilities. They should admit that they had failed to grow the cold virus and the place should be closed down.

Andrewes, naturally enough, did not agree, but this time the council had almost made up its mind. It placed the problem before its advisers on viruses and infections. I am not sure what swayed them but, after discussion, it decided to give the unit one more chance. Helio Pereira and Donna Chaproniere would take up new appointments, and if a suitable replacement medical virologist could be identified and would agree to come to the unit then it could have its life extended by another three years. But there were very few virologists in Britain at that time; nevertheless, someone had to be found if the work was to continue.

CHAPTER 5

A 'final' assault on the virus

I was the somewhat reluctant young virologist chosen for this one last effort to catch the virus, and I remember reflecting on how strange it was to find myself in such a position. Here I was being selected for this post and yet it was purely by force of circumstance that I became involved in the realm of virology at all. Having graduated in medicine at Sheffield I had originally been training to do clinical work. But that was in 1949 and all the intermediate training posts were being taken by demobilised doctors—quite rightly, in my view—while I had been rejected for military service. So the path I had originally set for myself was temporarily closed. However, my chief, Professor (later Sir) Charles Stuart-Harris, was a virologist as well as a clinician, and he offered me a job in his tiny research laboratory. I took it and entered the fascinating world of viruses. It was the start of a lifelong association.

I remained in Sheffield for nearly two years, working on the influenza virus, and then, in 1951, went to the Rockefeller Institute and Hospital in New York to do clinical work and continue learning research virology. It was an instructive period in which I was able to absorb current American thinking on the subject. It also confirmed my determination to work in this field. In 1954 I was invited back to Sheffield to run a new virus research laboratory under Stuart-Harris. In this period I studied adenovirus infections, poliovirus immunisation, and discovered a new virus—an enterovirus—that was causing an outbreak of meningitis and rash. This was getting really interesting and I could see my work in Sheffield extending far into the future. Or so I thought.

A call out of the blue

One day, less than three years later, Stuart-Harris casually mentioned that the secretary of the MRC would like to see me. This was how major events in a young scientist's career were handled in those days. Soon afterwards I found myself sitting in a deep armchair in a rather dark, old-style office in central London under the bright gaze of Sir Harold Himsworth, the dynamic head of the MRC. I had met him once before, but only briefly, when he was on a tour of inspection of my lab.

'Has Stuart-Harris told you what this is about?'

'No', I answered.

'Would you like to work at the Common Cold Research Unit?'

The question was quite unexpected and one that I certainly could not answer on the spur of the moment. Conflicting thoughts passed through my mind. Work had gone very well at Sheffield for the past two years and it would be a shame to stop. We had a house there and small children. This would be a big step into the unknown. I had visited the CCU and knew and respected Helio Pereira. But if Pereira had failed was I likely to succeed? No, I could not come to a decision right then.

I left saying I would think it over and discuss it with my wife. Interestingly he never mentioned that, in signing my contract of employment, I had agreed that I might be moved to another place of work.

After a great deal of heart-searching and much discussion I accepted the appointment, but it was understood that we would keep our house in Sheffield and if, after two years there was no sign of progress, we would go back. Stuart-Harris placed no obstacles in my path and agreed to release me. I discovered years later that he had suggested me for the post.

All Fools Day, April 1957, was chosen for our drive down to Wiltshire, a county I knew only vaguely. Our family, two adults and three small children plus a few personal possessions, were squeezed into a tiny Austin A30. The late afternoon weather was fine as we came slowly up the drive towards the main entrance of the CCU. But even the sunshine could not remove our feeling of dismay at what we saw: shabby green huts sprawled across the hilltop, presenting an uninviting image—not at all as I remembered it. This was more typical of some military establishments I had seen, and an unwelcome reminder of wartime conditions. In fact a Dutch colleague who visited us later said it looked just like the Nazi concentration camp in which he had suffered.

But these initial feelings were quickly forgotten in the warmth of our greeting. Welcoming staff met us at the top of the drive. And closer inspection showed that the huts were much nicer than they first appeared. They were spacious inside, warm, and centrally heated like our New York apartment. There was help for the mother and lots of places for the children to play. And the weather seemed milder and sunnier than in Sheffield. We soon settled in.

Encouraging a growth industry

By the time I walked into the lab I had already given much thought to what we should do. I still believed that the results of 1953 were valid. Of course the methods were complex and they had used a number of variable materials in their cultures. It seemed likely that they had, without knowing it, done everything right and perhaps been lucky with the cells they had used on that earlier occasion. In the repeat experiments they had probably changed something or, more likely, several things so that the virus could not grow. We would therefore start by using roller-tube cultures, just as they had done. This was the latest way of growing cells for virus work, and a method I had used a great deal in both New York and Sheffield.

The process involves taking a piece of tissue, such as kidney, cutting it into small segments and putting these into a solution of a digestive enzyme, trypsin. This loosens the cells from the fibres around them, allowing them to be separated by passing the mixture through a sterile gauze. The cells are then put into a nourishing solution, from which hundreds of test-tube cultures are produced. A test tube containing a small amount of this suspension is placed on its side in a warm place, causing the cells to stick to the glass and spread out. Tubes with fresh medium are

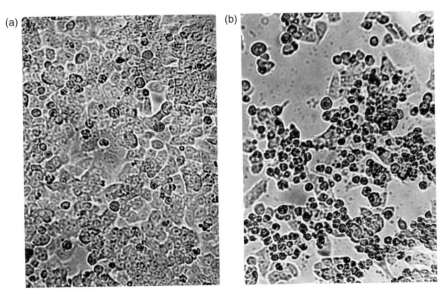

Fig. 5.1 A comparison between healthy and virus-infected cells. (a) A low-power, microscope view of a living culture of healthy human cells. The cells are normal, clear, and flat. (b) A similar culture that has been inoculated previously with a rhinovirus. The virus-infected cells have been killed and are round and dark, and readily float off the glass. They are easily recognised even though the virus particles are exceedingly small and only visible with the aid of an electron microscope.

placed in the roller drum in a warm cupboard (see Fig. 5.1), where they rotate slowly, causing them to experience alternate periods of exposure to air and then fluid to keep them healthy. If a virus is dropped into such a tube it attaches to the cells, starts growing in them, and will often kill them. It is quite easy to observe the cells through a simple microscope and see whether they have rounded up.

We would try out variants of the method, setting up a series of related but different cells and culture conditions that would enable us to test whether the virus would grow, even for a short while. When we found a method that worked to a limited extent we would change it little by little until we found a culture system in which virus would grow really well. Experiments would then be repeated regularly to make sure that the methods were reproducible. Others would then be able to grow the virus too.

But what cells to use? I had found in Sheffield that virtually any of the viruses we had would grow in human embryo kidney cells. Albert Sabin, the internationally famous microbiologist and developer of the live polio vaccine, visited us and said with great authority that any virus that grew in human kidney would grow in monkey kidney too.

A third suggestion came from John Enders. Having visited his lab in Boston I felt able to write to him and ask his advice. His reply, in a friendly and encouraging longhand airmail letter, recommended human amnion cells—something they were working on at the time. I thought we should use several different media too.

Next came the question of the environment in which to maintain the sample tubes? Physiology textbooks said the nose was cooler than the rest of the body. I used a thermocouple to check the temperature inside my nose and found it to be 33 °C rather than the 37 °C of deeper tissues. We would keep our roller drums in incubators at both temperatures. We could only guess at how fast the virus might grow and so decided to collect medium after three and then five days, periods in which the cells should remain healthy. Medium would also be taken from tubes without cells but inoculated with virus, and tubes with cells and medium but no virus. This would avoid our being misled by unknown viruses brought in with the cells or by traces of inoculated virus that had not disappeared.

Bring on the volunteers

So much thought was needed in those early stages: there were so many things we were uncertain about. But we had little time to spare. Volunteers were due to arrive the following week. It was time to stop theorising and get down to practice. We had less than five days and, at this point, no tissue culture or medium to test in them. It might be months before we could produce any. We needed a stock of an alternative virus and I preferred that it should not be the Donna Chaproniere virus that had caused so much trouble. Fortunately Pereira and his assistant Barbara Kelly had had colds just before they left and had taken nasal washings and left them in the deep freeze. I decided to accept their kind gift. The next thing was to plan what we were going to do with the 22 people we were expecting.

Our programme was quite simple. We would give each virus to a group of volunteers. And if they responded as expected, one in three of them would develop a cold. We could then wash out the noses of the volunteers and combine the washings to make a large pool, stored away in small amounts. From these we could dispense the same amount of virus to each of our range of tissue cultures. And we would have a stock of virus for our test-tube experiments.

It would be my first experience of infecting volunteers and giving them colds. Never before had I been given the chance of working with so many human guinea pigs. It was a wonderful opportunity, but how I wished I had time to give it more thought. In the past I had often spent weeks working out an experiment with one monkey or two rabbits, but not this time; and humans would be very different. Then I recalled the words of my chief in New York, Frank Horsfall, who said, 'Remember, Tyrrell, when it comes to an experiment, one human is worth the same as one mouse.' It seems a rather brutal statement from someone whom I knew to be a very humane person but, of course, in terms of their experimental and statistical value, he was quite correct. The important thing was to use sufficiently large numbers so that we could be sure of our results.

There was another matter to settle. This complicated programme of testing many different culture methods would generate dozens of samples of culture medium in the deep freeze. But it would take two weeks to test just one or two of them in volunteers. At that rate it would be years before we finished our first experiment. And we were planning quite a number. We had to shorten the procedure somehow.

The answer was to combine samples from a whole segment of the experiment and test the combined pool in volunteers. Provided we gave it to enough volunteers (8–10) we would be most unlikely to miss a positive pool. If the pool was negative we could say that the range of methods it represented was no good. If it worked we would test each of the constituents until we found which method had actually grown the virus.

It was a slow and boring work programme, and boring to read about. Research is like that: long periods of routine effort punctuated by frequent disappointments and the occasional success. But the high points make it all worthwhile. August 1957 saw us in one of the boring periods—we were just beginning our experiments. Monkey kidney cells were to be used at first, as recommended by Sabin. Human cells, in small numbers, would follow later.

The volunteers arrived on the Tuesday and waited the prescribed period so we could check that they had not brought any colds with them. At the end of the week they were inoculated with the pooled medium. It was vital to the success of the experiment that neither the person giving the inoculation nor the volunteer knew whether it was virus material or a dummy that was being dispensed. After the weekend a little charade was played out over morning coffee. I was one of the participants and the other was the medical superintendent, Dr M. L. (Bill) Bynoe.

Bill Bynoe was a fascinating example of the varied people we attracted. Born in the West Indies, he had studied medicine at St George's Hospital, London and then joined the Colonial Medical Service. He was captured during the Second World War and incarcerated in the notorious Changi Jail in Singapore, though his wife escaped to Australia. In spite of his experiences, he continued to work in Malaysia after the war but eventually retired to Britain. He was then persuaded to take on the role of medical superintendent at the CCU, where he quickly adapted to the research atmosphere, acting as a careful, clinical observer as well as a quiet and thorough administrator.

Bynoe, who did not know who had been given the virus, would say, in an apparently disinterested way, 'Oh, X in flat Y has got a cold.' I would sometimes know if the virus had been administered to that person but would act as if I did not, replying in an equally casual way, 'Oh, thank you. I must check in the lab to see what they had.' As our successes mounted this became ever more important.

And these first experiments were a success, but of a very tantalising sort. We did seem to produce good colds with culture fluids but the results would not repeat regularly, and testing the components took ages. There was evidence that virus would grow, but there were hints that the exact methods we used were important: human cells were better than monkey cells; 33 °C was better than 37 °C; and synthetic medium 199 was better than the rest. And if we attempted further passes from culture to culture, volunteer tests were negative. The virus died out.

A vote of confidence

It was at this stage that Sir Charles Harington came down to visit the lab and assess our progress. I was rather apologetic. A year had passed since my arrival but I could not really say we had found out how to grow the virus properly. But he seemed to be satisfied and obviously felt that we were beginning to get somewhere. I agreed with this assessment. It was true that we still had a long way to go but I now believed that we were making real progress and might eventually succeed. I felt less inclined to go back to Sheffield.

Our volunteer experiments showed that the virus would grow for a couple of passages but did not damage cells—or, at least, they appeared to be no different. We needed to continue our plan of changing the culture media step by step, but testing each variation by inoculating volunteers would be a very slow business. The process would be much shorter if we could develop alternative test-tube methods that would show when cells in a test tube were infected, even if they looked normal—a so-called *in vitro* or 'in glass' test-tube procedure. As luck would have it, two quite separate experiments provided us with the answer we were looking for.

In the past year we had been growing influenza viruses in tissue cultures of calf kidney cells to find out how viruses grow in cells and how to detect them. And it was during these experiments that I found evidence of virus interference—when a virus enters a cell and stops a second virus growing. This would enable us to detect a virus that does not kill cells. I also worked on a virus sent from Sweden as a candidate for the role of common cold virus. Known as the U-virus, it grew well in the kidney cells we used for our cold virus, causing cells to degenerate. We could easily measure the amount of virus formed because it agglutinated (stuck together) red cells.

I realised that we now had the elements we needed for an alternative test-tube method. If we combined what we had learned from these two studies we could put together a new procedure that would show when a cold virus was growing in our cells. So we set up cultures with cold virus in them and added the U-virus. A few days later we titrated the fluids and set about checking the results. The bench work was done by Griselda Worthington, an able young researcher who had trained as a biologist but subsequently developed an interest in viruses. She had given the culture fluids coded numbers. Then, to avoid bias, I read the results while she sat at the next bench and wrote down the figures on the experiment card. As we progressed her excitement grew. She could see there was far less U-virus in the cultures that had been given cold virus than in those that had not. The interference experiment had worked. It meant we could identify cultures infected with cold virus without having to give them to volunteers.

We now started altering the medium to protect the virus and make interference work even better. Gradually we achieved better interference and found that the cold virus would now pass from culture to culture as often as we wanted. It was a big step forward. Furthermore, we could prove that it was cold virus because, after, say, eight passages, the medium produced good colds in volunteers.

At this point Griselda had to leave the CCU and it seemed likely that research would be held up for want of skilled bench work. But Andrewes, with his usual speed off the mark, soon found a replacement. Using his network of contacts and with his customary lack of formality he invited Rosemary Parsons, a recent graduate from Bristol, to join us. She had been recommended by her professor, whom Andrewes knew. Trained as a microbiologist she had, like Griselda, a particular interest in viruses. Added to this was her love of the countryside and an interest in horse-riding.

Rosemary quickly became a valuable member of the team, helping to develop improved laboratory techniques and assisting in the first experiments to grow rhinoviruses.

Interference was not as convenient as the cell degeneration (cytopathic effect or CPE) seen with polio, but now that it was working we could make much better progress. Interference methods were used later to detect the rubella (German measles) virus in cells for the first time.

Disaster leads to success

Volunteer trials continued throughout the summer of 1959 because that was when people liked to come. They could get off work more easily and the weather was better. But we and our families also needed time off, and so lab work was reduced to a minimum for a few weeks. Nevertheless our recent success made me keen to get on with more interference experiments as soon as we returned.

More cells arrived and were distributed into medium and then into tubes. We waited eagerly for them to grow in the usual way but, when the day arrived to check on their progress, we were to meet with yet more disappointment. The results were awful. No beautiful clear cells spreading on the glass, just miserable rounded cells and the rubbish left by those that had died. What had gone wrong this time? I felt intensely frustrated. Our recent success had created a certain euphoria and I was keen to maintain this spirit. The problem had to be solved quickly.

The quickest method I could think of was to get ready-made and tested medium from the pharmaceutical laboratories. The drug firms were constantly

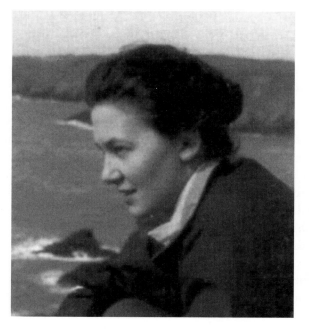

Fig. 5.2 Rosemary Parsons. (From Rosemary Hucker)

making and checking medium 199 for vaccine production, and we believed
it gave the best results. It was an American development with scores of ingredients, from sugars to vitamins. So I rang round my friends in the industry
explaining, 'Something awful has happened to our medium. Please send me
some of yours—not just the basic medium but all the things we add to it. I'm
not even sure we can produce distilled water any more.' They cooperated
splendidly and soon medium arrived from three different laboratories. Cells
arrived too, and we decided to try all the media. We used them exactly as they
were sent, even though the medium from Glaxo Laboratories looked too
acidic—it apparently added less sodium bicarbonate than we did.

This time all went well: all the cells in all the tubes with all the media looked
fine. Rather than waste them we decided to repeat the interference experiment
and added HGP (the cold virus left us by Helio Pereira) to some of the
cultures growing in each medium. But a few days later something seemed to
have gone wrong. Cell degeneration (CPE), like that produced by U-virus,
had occurred in some of the tubes. Could I have put the wrong virus into
them? A few more tests showed that there was no mix-up. In fact things had
turned out better than we could have hoped. The interference test we had

been using was no longer needed. In the tubes with the Glaxo medium the virus had grown so well that it had killed the cells just as the U-virus did. Further investigation showed that the higher acidity of this particular medium was the reason.

This was wonderful news. Not only had we overcome the medium problem very quickly but we had also identified an important component leading to success in growing cold viruses. In order to detect the HGP virus in a nasal washing all we had to do was to inoculate it into our new type of culture, and in about five days time the cells would degenerate in a typical way. All this work would make a really good scientific paper. But we must be careful. Common cold research was full of reports on methods of growing viruses that other people could not confirm. So we sent our results and some materials to friendly virologists: Geoffrey Schild, working for Stuart-Harris in Sheffield, and Peggy Pereira, now at the Virus Reference Laboratory at Colindale. They repeated the experiments and confirmed what we said. We now felt ready to publish and sent off a three-part paper to *The Lancet*, who speedily accepted and published it in January 1960.

It was quite a landmark and a considerable boost to our confidence. It also meant that we were able to bring in more bright young scientists to exploit the situation and intensify our research into the new viruses. One of these was Dr Nigel Dimmock, whose enthusiasm for science was aroused at an early age and led first to a degree in zoology at Liverpool University and then to a PhD at Reading University while working at the CCU. It was here that he did some of the first work on the physical properties of rhinovirus particles. Subsequently he went to Canberra, Australia for postdoctoral experience and then returned to the new University of Warwick. Now a professor, he has acquired an international reputation for his work on how antibodies neutralise viruses.

Perhaps the most important result of all this work was that it made it possible to start thinking about colds in the way we did with other infections. I remember walking down the drive one evening, feeling quite excited and wondering where we might go from here. We could measure antibodies now and find out if people develop immunity. We could collect viruses and work out if there are different types, as there are with polio. We could make a vaccine and see if it would protect. We might even be able to study the structure of the virus and find out how it was able to multiply in cells.

I came down to earth in the end. But much of my thinking was perfectly reasonable, though what we actually found was more varied and more surprising than I could possibly have imagined.

The heart of the matter

Whilst scientists like myself were hunting viruses or trying to make vaccines, others were penetrating ever more deeply into the structure of the human body, trying to identify the basic components of a living cell and how these relate to each other. This work went on in what seemed like ivory-tower centres and, though most biologists did not realise it at the time, it was about to revolutionise our ideas concerning life in all its forms—from human bodies to viruses.

I think it came home to me most forcefully in January 1957, just before I moved to Salisbury. I had been invited back to New York City to attend a meeting in honour of Basil O'Connor, the great polio activist. This time I was to fly the Atlantic. The plane was old and propeller-driven and would have to make several stops to refuel—once it got going, that is. At the last moment it was found to be faulty and so, after some delay, BOAC took us on a long coach ride to a hotel for the night. We were told we would have to share rooms, causing each of us to look around for someone we knew at least a little. It transpired that the only person I had met before was a certain Dr Francis Crick, also employed by the MRC. And so we agreed to share.

Crick was already famous for his work with James Watson showing that, in DNA crystals, the molecules are arranged as spirals with the nucleotides linked together as mirror image pairs. It would be nice to record that we talked far into the night on scientific matters, but it was late, we were tired and, as I recall, we talked only a little, and then not about science. In the morning we split up and were taken, like packages on a conveyor belt, to the airport and New York.

Basil O'Connor was a friend of Franklin Roosevelt and, through his influence, had spent thirty years in promoting and funding research on poliomyelitis through the 'March of Dimes' and in other ways. As a central part of the meeting there was a programme of scientific papers under the aegis of the New York Academy of Science. Firstly we heard the latest news on the development and testing of the new killed and live vaccines against poliomyelitis, based on old-style virus methods. Then we heard that the poliovirus had been thoroughly purified and saw electron microscope pictures and details of its chemical composition to prove it.

The meeting then changed gear: Francis Crick appeared on the podium and was listened to with great attention, particularly by other experts in his subject. He spoke as a crystallographer, describing with pictures of X-ray diffraction (scattering) patterns why the strands of DNA in crystals had to be arranged in the form of the double helix that he and James Watson had described in 1953. Watson and Crick, later to be awarded the Nobel Prize, had

Better media coverage

During those post-war years the general laboratory facilities we had in Britain compared unfavourably with those enjoyed by our friends in the USA. Our problems with the virus growth medium were an example of this. It was customary at that time for virus labs to make their own media in the 'media kitchen'; but it took a long time and the resulting fluids were often of no use, usually because of minor glitches which took ages to detect and put right. Tiny traces of impurity or a chemical flaw in a single ingredient—out of the dozens needed—meant that the cells would no longer grow or even survive. The human cells would grow well only in very high-quality fluid media. Pharmaceutical laboratories helped us out for a while, but it would have been unfair to rely upon their goodwill for more than a limited period. Help, fortunately, was at hand.

A young postdoctoral member of the unit, Paul Chapple, would prove instrumental in solving this media problem. Having studied microbiology at Bristol University and then acquired a PhD degree, he had been recruited by Andrewes to join in laboratory studies of the new rhinoviruses. He quickly adapted to life at the CCU, combining his research work with a keen interest in amateur photography. In fact his skills in the latter were sufficient for his films of volunteer life and the new methods of organ culture to be awarded prizes by the local photographic society. Then came the move which was to be so beneficial to us—he left to set up a UK branch of the American firm Flow Laboratories and make tissue culture materials commercially.

Suddenly we were able to buy media made to a high standard, and one of our biggest headaches disappeared almost overnight. Of course it cost money, but it saved us so much in staff time wasted on making and testing small amounts of medium and on doing experiments that failed. At first we had difficulty in explaining these extra costs to our financial masters but they eventually came round to our way of thinking.

Chapple later moved to the USA to do similar work, for a while becoming director of the Alton Jones Cell Science Center in Lake Placid, NY, and later an independent consultant.

In the USA, labs like ours were able to buy not just media but complete batches of grown cultures ready for inoculation. They had money and there were firms able to do the job. It was one reason that they were able to carry out such large-scale studies. These kits have developed much further since those early days, and it is now normal for laboratories throughout the world to do their work using very complex and carefully standardised biological reagents and 'test kits' prepared commercially.

Communications

The unavailability of a product in this country would not be such a disadvantage nowadays when items can be ordered by telephone, email, or on the internet, and then air-freighted from almost anywhere in the world in little more than a day. But we are talking about a time when travel across the Atlantic was more frequently undertaken by boat than by plane, and our main methods of communication were post and a very basic telephone system.

Letters offered a reliable and fairly quick method by the standards of the time, at least within the UK. And we had telephone lines to the outside world. Internally we employed the services of a telephone switchboard, an impressive affair of large, red jack-plugs that were pushed into labelled sockets on a huge panel that loomed over the operator. It may have been a dinosaur but it was durable and enabled people to send messages around the site and for volunteers to be connected with distant friends and relatives. Late in the 1980s it was replaced, and much sought after by museums.

The performance of the telephone system improved steadily over the years. At first international calls were expensive and had to be booked, and the voices were often almost unintelligible: so bad that we continued to use letters as far as possible. An airmail letter to the USA would get a reply in about ten days, and for a great many matters involved in our joint research this was fast enough. Telephone was fine for enquiring or ordering from people in our vicinity.

By the 1980s we could dial anywhere and make immediate contact, and the sound quality was so good you could not tell whether the speaker was a few miles away or on the other side of the world. The telephone culture had arrived, though we were still lagging behind the USA.

Letters and telephones served us well but in matters of science, as in many other disciplines, there is no substitute for face-to-face meetings. These are an essential part of scientific life. I attended many meetings and conferences over the years and found them invaluable as a means of finding out what was really going on and discussing concepts and difficulties. Initially I went to these international meetings and the laboratories of others working in my field by sea and land but, of course, this eventually gave way to air travel.

Not an exact science

Scientific research is one of the more nebulous branches of human activity: its scope for variation is endless, its outcome uncertain. Science and our approach to it are constantly changing. People move on and others take over. And as the science changed so did the administration and funding. A more controlled approach became evident. Official channels were now used for recruitment, replacing the more casual approach described earlier. Everyday life was changing, and the CCU had to adjust to this and to the new ideas in science.

It is notoriously difficult to predict how new lines of discovery will develop. Even commercially directed research, such as drug development, can be full of surprises. The government view in the 1970s was that medical research would be more successful and give more useful results if it were directed towards the health problems of the nation. And they commissioned Lord Rothschild to write a report to show how this could be done. In it he enunciated a customer–contractor principle. The idea was that customers, in this case the health departments, say what they want to be discovered and provide money for the contractor, in this case the MRC, to do the job. This contrasted with general MRC policy, which was to find talented people in a general area that seemed promising for development and support the individual to do his or her best.

It could be argued that setting up the CCU and directing research there, with colds identified as a national problem, was anticipating Lord Rothschild by a few decades. But quick results were impossible to achieve, because so much important enabling research had still to be done.

The best investigators, and the most successful, will wait until the time is ripe before they tackle a health problem. They look for that moment when knowledge has advanced sufficiently and appropriate methods have become available. Then they have both a clear objective and the means by which to achieve it.

So what is the best form of research? Should we be pursuing blue sky (fundamental) research or concentrate on goal-directed or applied research? The argument has continued for as long as I can remember, and both viewpoints are strongly supported. But the truth is that both can be done well or badly and that both need and support each other. Louis Pasteur provides an example in support of the former. As a chemist he was investigating why wine went bad and discovered the microbes that spoiled it. And while doing this he also discovered stereo-isomerism—molecules and crystals that are mirror images of each other. The history of science is full of such chance findings.

Sir Harold Himsworth visualised medical knowledge as a sphere with organisms and diseases at the surface, while inside lay the causes and the mechanisms which brought them about. An example is the paralysis of the deficiency disease, beriberi—the symptom on the surface. Just inside the sphere was the knowledge that this was due to lack of vitamin B_1. Deeper still was the knowledge that the vitamin was part of the cell's machinery for producing energy through enzymes and other molecules.

The story of common colds corresponds with this view: a full understanding includes knowledge ranging from recognising symptoms and human behaviour to the way the protein on the surface of a virus is arranged; and how an antibody or a drug can slot into its surface. It is rather like peeling away the layers of an onion in order to probe deeper as each successful piece of research exposes further underlying mysteries to which an answer must be found.

Looking for winners

Official consensus or community views may help or hinder the process of rating or ranking problems and targets of research or development. I remember it being pointed out that the Department of Health could not do anything about a particular problem—developing and appointing specialists in infections—until the profession saw a need for action. Similarly, pharmaceutical companies may look at a new science that suggests new possibilities for treatment, but will not undertake development unless there is also the potential for sales that will cover their costs and yield dividends for the shareholders. If they get it wrong, then the resultant losses will have to be covered by the sales of other, more profitable products. I still recall the impact of a remark by a very able research worker in the commercial sector: 'Remember, David, no one pays us to do research the way the taxpayer pays for yours. Our ability to do research is directly related to our product earnings.'

New science, even potentially exciting new science pointing to new medications, is not sufficient incentive on its own. There has to be a convergence of interests which causes the matter to be placed high on the agenda of several groups, and then things will start to happen.

I was well aware that the continuance of our particular line of research was dependent upon the goodwill of a number of people, in the MRC in particular, who had been extraordinarily patient over many years. Throughout this long period of research they had given us physical support and salaries, and reviewed these at regular intervals. But on what basis was the decision taken to continue? The project had to be worthwhile of course but, beyond that, it seems they placed most importance on that intangible: the quality of the individual. The people they rated highly were, obviously, intelligent, but they might be loners or gregarious; orderly or untidy; constantly throwing out ideas, arguing and doing new experiments or quietly and carefully developing their thoughts; and they might like new and complex methods or be content to work with the old and simple. There was (and is) no standard format for a good investigator. Nevertheless Harold Himsworth said that the people they supported usually knew all about the detail and technology of their particular subject (say a disease or a type of biology), but would also have picked up the basic ideas and recent advances in other medical and biological fields.

We were remarkably fortunate with the people that we attracted to the CCU. Many of them achieved considerable eminence in their chosen fields, but this could only be guessed at when they started. Quite industrious students do not necessarily retain this quality as they mature. Real ability could only be shown once they were operating in an environment which suited them. The system relied substantially on an ability to choose people well, arrange a suitable placement, and then support them for some years in a research group or under an experienced investigator. Successful research depended on building teams with the right mix of talent and experience. Ultimately, people were judged by results, and if after several years they had not produced novel, published work, then they would not be reappointed. A certain amount of luck might be involved—being in the right place at the right time, possibly accompanied by a fortunate breakthrough.

The parts they played

In a book like this it is only possible to tell part of the story of common cold studies in the UK, let alone in the world as a whole. As a result it may appear that most of the work was done by a rather small group of investigators. This is far from true. We benefited from the loyal collaboration of a wide variety of people. Some spent much of their lives at the CCU. For others it was just a stage in their careers, and they moved on; quite a number of them achieving high positions in the academic world. Inevitably there was a high proportion of men amongst the senior researchers, simply because there were far more men in science at the time. But it was by no means a male preserve. Many gifted women joined us, some staying for long periods, and were involved in crucial areas of the research. Some were highly qualified before they came, others continued their studies while at the CCU.

One example of the latter was Kathy Brown. Brought up in Salisbury and a product of the local South Wilts Grammar School for Girls, she had a strong interest in natural history and did well in her science exams. Since the unit was one of the few places locally where she could pursue this interest in science, she applied to join us directly from school. Beginning as technician to Helio Pereira, Kathy then took courses in medical technology and passed all the exams of the Institute of Medical Laboratory Technicians, eventually obtaining their fellowship with a thesis based on one of her research projects.

In a few years she had risen to be chief technician with responsibility for handling the tissue culture work. Kathy Brown's personal qualities made her particularly suited to this work—someone who generated a friendly atmosphere amongst those around her and took scrupulous care in all laboratory procedures. I do not think the unit could have managed without her.

Another recruit from the same grammar school came to us and found romance. Pam Ball joined immediately upon completing her secondary education and was given basic training in our laboratory. She then worked as a technician with Brigadier Buckland, who features later in our story. The object of her affections, 'Brad' Bradburne, worked here as a PhD student and stayed until he received his doctorate. He took a post at Wellcome Research, and they married and raised a family nearby. This happy ending was not untypical, for the unit brought a number of couples together over the years. And, like so many others, Pam kept in contact with the CCU long after she had left.

An interesting contrast was Beverly Head, who also grew up locally but left school with few qualifications. Some might have thought this an obstacle to joining the CCU but Bev, as she was known, was determined that cold research was what she wanted to do. Her enthusiasm at interview won the day and she was taken on. A good bench worker, she took no exams but played a particular role in looking after the collection of viruses and other materials that we held for WHO, producing and testing these, assisting visiting WHO scientists, and, later, collecting and processing the daily specimens from volunteers. An interest in local affairs developed and she eventually became mayor of Salisbury.

Memories of that time naturally focus on those involved in research, but there were many others whose job it was to look after the people who were housed and fed and lived their lives there. Some of these are remembered not because of what they did but because of what they were, and because of the wholehearted way in which they performed their particular tasks. Over the years the CCU played host to a rich and varied selection of such people.

One of these was known to all and sundry simply as Miss Rae, and her job was vital. She was the cook—and a very good one. Having served in the war she came to us immediately upon demobilisation. Erect in posture and with a serious expression, she produced generous home-style meals for volunteers and resident staff; even preparing special gluten-free dishes when one of my daughters required a special diet. At the same time she cared for an aged mother who lived on the site with her. Miss Rae stayed until retirement age, and even then we did not want her to go.

Another who will be remembered, particularly by the volunteers, was Audrey Rogers. Brought up and educated locally, she joined us only after she had married and raised a family. Her job, officially, was to help in the linen room, but her outgoing and friendly nature inevitably led her into taking on a number of hospitality functions: shopping for the volunteers in town, finding them Wellington boots for country walks, and generally making their stay as pleasant as possible. She became their constant friend in need.

Denis the gardener was another whose contribution to the folklore of the unit lingers in the mind. His path to the CCU was somewhat unusual—he had been trained in gardening while a patient at a local mental hospital. Having recovered, he came to tend the grounds of the unit and succeeded in softening the prison camp aspect somewhat. Easily spotted by his shock of brown hair and constant activity, he made use of odd corners of the site to raise plants and then set these out to produce colourful summer displays. His standards were so high that the unit received awards in the annual 'Britain in Bloom' competitions. It also emerged, to the surprise of many, that he was a great lover of Shakespeare and could quote at length from his works.

Others stood out because of the dedication they brought to their work. Typical of these was Hilda Andrews who grew up on an outlying farm in the area. As a young woman she took a job as a maid, working under the matron and with the other domestic staff to ensure that the flats were always spotless and well cared for. A need to look after ageing parents took her away for a spell and then she returned, to stay until retirement. Always busy, Hilda found time to serve as a church organist at Stratford-sub-Castle, on the edge of Salisbury, cycling some eight to ten miles each Sunday to attend. And even in retirement, still cheerful and smiling though seriously disabled, she continued to keep the rooms in her old cottage up to 'Harvard' standards.

Meeting expectations

Businesses, if they are at all successful, constantly monitor the work of individual departments, and research organisations need to adopt similar measures if they are to ensure that their resources are being properly used. Our work was reviewed at intervals but never in any oppressive way. Having elected to support a particular project, the general policy was to let the people concerned get on with the job without looking over their shoulders every few months. As I suggested earlier, the outcome of research is unpredictable and rarely produces results as quickly as one hopes at the outset. Our meetings gave us an opportunity to discuss the progress of our work. We were also expected to send in copies of all published papers, because this indicated

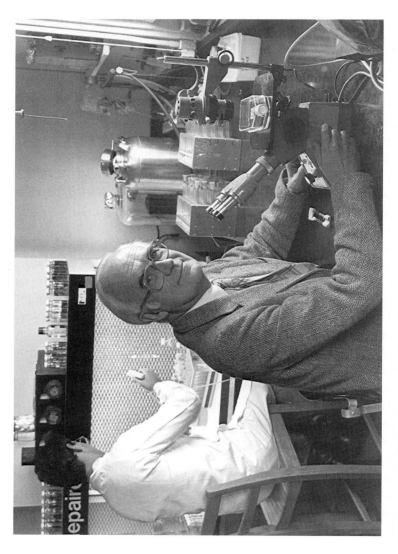

Fig. 5.4 Part of the CCU laboratory: David Tyrrell is seen checking cells on the surface of a plastic bottle by means of a binocular microscope; behind him a technician is pipetting in a cabinet supplied with filtered, sterile air; to the right are stainless steel tanks for preserving cells chilled by liquid nitrogen; and in front of those are test tubes in which cells settle onto a glass surface.

that work we had done had been looked at by fellow scientists, who thought well of it. And we summarised our main research for an annual report.

The most detailed review of the operation and scientific output of the unit took place at intervals of a few years when the MRC sent a committee of experts to study our work at close hand. I was happy with this pattern but the visits were stressful. Written accounts of our research were prepared, and when the committee arrived we had to arrange for staff members to give talks on their work and answer any questions that the visitors raised. Sometimes we could gauge what the committee was thinking, but the crucial question was what would its written report say and what would the council decide after it had seen it? I knew that if the MRC was dissatisfied the unit would be closed. But each time it seemed we had done enough to suggest that it should continue to support us.

Our budget covered the programme of cold research which we had agreed with the council but there were times when we saw advantages in going beyond the boundaries that had been set. Then we usually needed more funds. I can recall, on one occasion, when we had high hopes of gaining approval for a particular project and then found that, through no fault of our own, we had got our timing wrong. As anyone involved in applying for funds will know this is often the most crucial element. In this case it was not a question of more money for our research but a matter of improving the housing in which this research took place. Our buildings at the unit, only intended as temporary, were in a poor state of repair and it was suggested that we replace them with brick constructions. This was to be done in such a way that, once we had finished with them, they could be converted easily to another use—perhaps flats or a geriatric home. The idea had been suggested by a visiting committee.

Our director, Sir Christopher Booth, and I were invited to a council meeting at which the proposed scheme was to be discussed. We had taken a lot of time in preparing our proposal and employed professional help from architects, surveyors, etc. We were optimistic as we arrived at the meeting room in the head office at Park Crescent and were placed at one end of a long, polished table at which all the council members were seated. The signs were good. The project had been initiated by the MRC and so was clearly something it wanted. We had carefully prepared all the necessary costing. It promised to be a fairly routine, rubber-stamping operation. But we reckoned without government intervention. On that very day the MRC had received instructions to cut a substantial amount of money from its expenditure. And as our project was valued at a figure similar to the reduction requested, it was clear to the meeting that it could solve its problem at a stroke by not voting for the rebuilding.

All we received was some money for paint and materials for minor building repairs.

Someone has to pay for it

Research requires a lot of money and other resources. I do not know how early research on colds was funded: the early tests on bacterial vaccines may have been paid for in fees to the laboratory who made them up and administered them. Walter Kruse, when conducting his cold research in 1913 and 1914, was running an institute in an established medical school in Leipzig. The two experiments he carried out were so small and simple that he could probably have paid any expenses out of his departmental funds. In spite of this neither he nor anyone else in his department continued the studies after the war. They concentrated instead on bacterial and gastrointestinal infections, and on the welfare and nutrition of children. These would have been more in line with his earlier research and more relevant to the needs of the local community and government.

Alphonse Dochez was based in the medical school of Columbia University in New York City. He would certainly have needed substantial funds to provide isolation rooms for animals and humans within the hospital. Some of the work was supported by The Chemical Foundation Inc., and there were other sources as well. As Dochez's work became better known it must have attracted even more sponsorship. Remarkably, in spite of his success, he left cold research and moved into basic studies of bacteria. Later, at the Rockefeller Institute, he wrote with Oswald Avery the paper that showed that DNA carried the genes of bacteria.

In the early 1930s senior people in the MRC had talked to colleagues in the USA about Dochez's work and were glad to support an attempt to confirm it in Britain. But these years of the Great Depression demanded rigid economy in research, as in every other sphere throughout the nation. When Andrewes was given only £200 to cover the cost of an extra clinical colleague for six months it was clearly insufficient for the whole project, and the balance had to come out of his laboratory budget at the NIMR.

In Britain the work of the CCU was supported by the MRC and Ministry of Health while national and some local surveys were paid for by the Public Health Laboratory Service. And a few smaller organisations made grants. Drug firms would also offer help, but this was frowned upon in the early days. I remember when one of them wanted to provide us with some water baths, presumably having noticed the age of the ones we were using. I went to see the director of the NIMR, Sir Charles Harington about it, but he was emphatically opposed. 'You certainly can't accept anything, Tyrrell. The MRC is relied upon by the Government as an independent adviser. If it was realised in the House that the unit had accepted money from industry, questions would certainly be asked and our advice would no longer be trusted.'

But attitudes change

Attitudes began to alter in the 1960s. The MRC wanted to avoid accusations that it had failed to prevent other countries from making money out of the discovery of interferon (see Chapter 11). This seemed to have the potential to become as important an antiviral drug as penicillin had been in the past. So they entered into agreements with drug firms to have a joint interferon committee to develop the drug, obtain patent protection, and share any royalties that came along. There were none. The development work was far more difficult and slower than anyone could have foreseen at the time. The links with the other interested and capable laboratories were enjoyable and helpful, but so were many other such links in which there was no formal or commercial bond.

Attitudes continued to change and, by the 1980s, MRC staff were being allowed to accept grants from outside bodies, on certain conditions. In our case trials of drugs had become much more complicated and laborious and therefore more costly, and money was tight within the MRC. So when the time came for a drug trial with volunteers, the full cost of such a trial at the unit was calculated and the firm involved would pay half. This put us on an equal footing with the drug developers, and we only took on those trials which we considered would contribute to our overall scientific programme. In addition we could be involved in developing treatments for the viruses we had discovered. There was no group within the MRC doing such work so their help was essential to us. But they, in turn, needed results from our volunteers.

In this way we could not be accused of being 'bought' by industry and having our programme dictated or dominated by them. Indeed we did on occasion refuse to do studies which would not have contributed to our overall plans. Collaborative studies were also conducted with academic groups in universities and other institutions, where no money changed hands.

This greater freedom was particularly helpful when we took an interest in the psychological aspects of colds. American funds enabled us to pay for extra staff, buy new computers, and carry out studies with Carnegie Mellon

University without impairing the work we were already doing on the treatment and biology of colds. Similar changes took place in the USA: for example the armed forces gave grants to the group at Charlottesville for epidemiological studies of colds. But later on their projects were funded by pharmaceutical laboratories. And universities and research organisations gave underlying support by providing facilities and an environment in which research could be carried out (See chapters nine and eleven).

A number of factors come into play when determining how research and development are to be financed. What is the nature of the work, who is doing it, what are the attitudes and perceptions of the time, and what are the policies and purposes of the fund provider? It follows that a great deal of future clinical and scientific change will depend upon its appeal to those who have the money to support it.

CHAPTER 6

Viruses and their targets

There has been much confusion concerning viruses and bacteria and what, if any, are the differences between them. This is not surprising since even the scientists who first studied them shared this confusion. But the differences are fundamental. A bacterium is self-sufficient. It can survive on its own without any exterior aid and multiply rapidly through cell division. A virus is essentially parasitic. It can do nothing on its own and becomes active only after it has penetrated a living cell. Once inside it produces more viruses, often destroying the host cell and then going on to attack adjacent cells. It is the type of virus and the type of cell it attacks which determines the nature of any disease which follows.

Viruses are very 'clever', being able to adapt rapidly to changing conditions, but so is the body. It is by no means a foregone conclusion that a virus attack will lead inevitably to some form of illness. We are involved with viruses all the time. Some viruses live inside our bodies from childhood to old age and either cause no illness or only occasional problems like cold sores. We swallow or breathe in other viruses, and more often than not they do us no harm. Even if they infect us for a while our immune system is very good at getting rid of them. Some people are attacked more than others, but our bodies win the battle on most occasions.

Another big difference between bacteria and viruses is size. Bacteria can be studied and identified with an optical microscope. Viruses are many thousands of times smaller and so remained invisible until modern technology brought vastly increased levels of magnification through the electron microscope. Cold viruses vary in size but, on average, several hundred thousand of them would fit comfortably on a pinhead. If you placed the smallest of them, the rhinoviruses, side by side then you would need some 2400 to equal the width of one human hair.

Perhaps a more graphic analogy would be to imagine that if a single rhinovirus particle could be enlarged to the size of a golf ball and your body increased its size in proportion then you could sleep with your head in England and your feet somewhere in the Mediterranean. Translated to the USA this could mean having the sounds of Broadway ringing in your ears while dipping your toes in the Gulf of Mexico.

We do not know how many different viruses there are, except that their number probably runs into thousands. An accurate count is impossible because many viruses modify themselves when the need arises, making it difficult both to classify and to combat them. They invade all classes of living organisms—bacteria, fungi, plants, and animals—causing, in humans, such diseases as chickenpox, smallpox, poliomyelitis, yellow fever, herpes, AIDS, Lassa fever, Ebola, influenza, and the common cold. In domestic animals they are responsible for foot and mouth disease, swine fever, rabies, and canine distemper. Each disease is associated with a particular family of viruses that target specific types of cells, each virus employing its own peculiar chemical and genetic strategies. Although these families share certain features there are also substantial differences between them. And even within each family there are numerous variations in species, their shape, and their size.

Nowadays anyone can tell you that there are a couple of hundred cold viruses, and they may well know something about them belonging to different families. Those are the elementary facts but they still represent more than I or anyone else knew when common cold research started up after the Second World War. At that time the best-informed virologist could say 'a virus can cause a cold in human beings'; and if he was wise (it would have to be 'he', there were no female virologists studying colds then) he would say no more. The viruses that had been identified up to that point were detected because they caused an illness such as smallpox or poliomyelitis. They were distinguishable from bacteria because they would pass through the usual filters used for removing bacteria; and they would only grow in the presence of living cells, while bacteria would grow in non-living media—soups and jellies.

What makes a virus?

These criteria did not in fact separate what we now call true viruses from some small bacteria, and as a result led to real confusion. Viruses were identified essentially by what they did, the diseases they caused, and not by what they were. In fact if they didn't make something sick—an animal, a plant, or a bacterium—then we could not be aware of their existence. Experiments with improved filters had shown, before the war, that viruses were either particles or firmly stuck to them. Only in the 1940s were electron microscopes good enough to make virus particles clearly visible. And even then it was difficult to distinguish between a small number of particles and the junk from dead cells. The problem was in getting enough virus and purifying it from all the other material in a cell. Many people were not at all sure that virus particles had ever been seen. It was safer to think of them as some vague fluid, perhaps a special protein of some sort.

We now know that a virus particle is an extremely simple form of life, having only two main components: a piece of nucleic acid, RNA or DNA, and a protective protein shell that surrounds it. The nucleic acid is the infectious part of the virus. It also contains the genetic information which determines its characteristics.

Nucleic acids consist of sugar molecules joined together by phosphate in repeated patterns to form long chain compounds which are coiled up in the interior of the virus particle (see Fig. 6.1). Depending on whether the sugars are ribose or deoxyribose, the resultant nucleic acid will be either RNA (ribonucleic acid) or DNA (deoxyribonucleic acid). A ribose molecule is a ring containing a chain of five carbon atoms and a deoxyribose has one less side chain on it. So all virus particles contain at least one strand of DNA or RNA, but never both. These carry the information needed to make the protein, the other essential constituent of a virus particle.

The information is carried by ring-shaped molecules containing nitrogen which occur as single (pyrimidine) or double (purine) rings, and only two of each sort are used. These are attached at intervals to the sugars, rather like charms on a bracelet (see Fig. 6.1c), and the sugar molecules are linked together by phosphate groups. Each unit of the chain is known as a nucleotide, and it is the order in which they are strung together that spells out the genetic information which gives each virus its unique character. A group of three nucleotides in a particular sequence, known as a codon, forms a unit in the genetic code and specifies which amino acid is to be incorporated into a certain protein; a series of codons will then identify the complete protein. The mechanism has been likened to a series of 'letters' written in a code which then determines not only the amino acid content of the protein but also other cell functions.

Proteins are built from amino acids, and their type, quantity, and sequence determine the way in which they behave. They may join up to form a membrane, or coil into a tough ball, or bind tightly to some other part of the cell—or to the fats and sugars it contains. Some proteins are enzymes which act as catalysts to cut molecules apart or to join them together. The 'triplet code', with minor variations, applies throughout the living world and is 'written' with only a handful of nucleotides. Yet it can direct the assembly of 20 or so amino acids to form thousands of different proteins, which determine the structure and function of everything from plants and animals to bacteria and viruses. It is an astonishing concept.

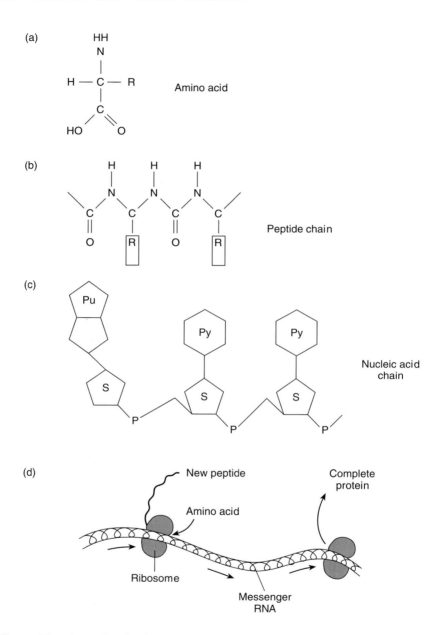

Fig. 6.1 (a) Amino acid molecules are built up from individual atoms of hydrogen (H), nitrogen (N), carbon (C), and oxygen (O), linked together in a chain. Each molecule contains a further side chain, the R group, which determines the properties of that particular amino acid. There are over 100 different types. (b) Amino acid molecules will link together in long chains—the amino group of one joining to the acid group of another—to form proteins. The properties of these proteins will depend upon the particular amino acids from which they are

New viruses for old

Procreation is the name of the game. A virus, like any other life form, only survives if it perpetuates the species. But, left to itself, it lacks the necessary equipment. The only way it can succeed is by invading some more advanced organism and making use of its resources, perverting them to suit its own requirements. We can follow the process by looking at how one of the simpler viruses, a rhinovirus, multiplies. This particular virus has an RNA gene inside a fairly rigid protein capsule. If we breathe it in it will attack the cells in the nose. Figure 6.2 illustrates the process diagrammatically.

The protein sticks to particular patches on the surface of some cells, and this triggers the cell to form a dip which becomes a pocket and then a little balloon. Once inside the cell the capsule opens up and the RNA is released. It finds itself in the jelly of the cell where there are amino acids and what are known as transfer molecules whose function is to move the amino acids about. The virus now sets about replicating itself so that it can attack other cells. Its single RNA strand joins the RNA strands of the host cell which are carrying the messages to make normal cell proteins. The transfer molecules are now fooled into bringing the amino acids to the foreign virus RNA, and it quickly strings these together to form a long protein chain. The first step of the invasion has succeeded.

---

formed and the sequence in which they are linked together. (c) Nucleic acids determine the genetic characteristics of the virus. They consist of pyrimidine (Py) and purine (Pu) molecules containing rings of carbon and nitrogen atoms linked by phosphate groups—single rings in the case of pyrimidine and double rings in the case of purine. The diagram shows the molecular structure with rings of pyrimidine and purine, a sugar molecule (S) with five carbon atoms, and the phosphate link (P), which together form the nucleic acid. New nucleic acids are formed through the action of an enzyme—a polymerase—that copies a strand by adding new units to form a double chain alongside it. However, this copy is a 'negative' since each purine is copied with a pyrimidine and each pyrimidine with purine. This is because the two units, or nucleotides, fit together very well and make a paired chain of an even width. If the negative is copied again then a 'positive' chain is formed which has exactly the same pattern as the first. (d) The 'recipe' or information on how to make a protein is written, or encoded, in strands of nucleic acid, with each amino acid identified by a codon (a sequence of three nucleotides). The coded message is revealed through a process called 'translation', illustrated here. A ribosome particle—a beautifully constructed ball of nucleic acid and protein—attaches to the starting point of a positive strand of RNA (often called a messenger). It then runs quickly along it, pausing briefly to 'read' the coded message. In response to each codon the ribosome takes up a different amino acid from the many with which it is surrounded in the jelly of the cell and joins this onto the last amino acid it picked up, immediately going on to read the next letters of the message. When it reaches a special 'stop' codon, the protein chain is released and moves on to be further processed.

Part of this long protein forms an enzyme that cuts the chain at specific points and the pieces then start to behave independently. One group forms another large enzyme molecule (a polymerase) and this sets about replicating the virus RNA strand, which it does in two stages. First the enzyme takes nucleotides from the cell and links them to form a negative copy. And from this it produces exact positive replicas. Meanwhile the rest of the original long protein is forming into a shell made from distinct proteins which then

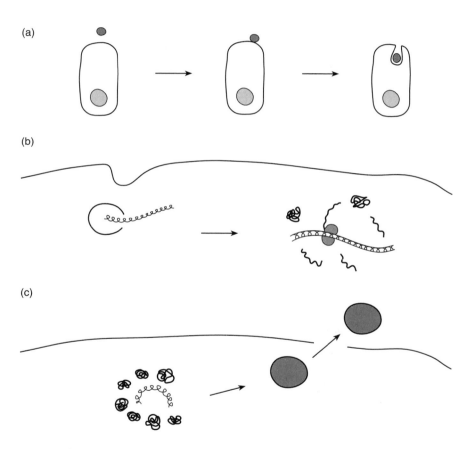

Fig. 6.2 The growth of a virus, based on the growth of the very simplest of common cold viruses, the rhinoviruses. (a) A virus particle is carried to the surface of a cell, attaches to it, and is taken in. (b) The nucleic acid comes out of the virus particle. This is translated into protein, including enzymes to make more nucleic acid and other proteins for building the outside of more particles. (c) Protein molecules collect around a new strand of positive RNA and form a shell for new particles. The cell is damaged and degenerates and new particles are shed.

surround the new RNA strand. The process is complete—a fresh infectious particle has been formed. This is repeated thousands or millions of times, resulting in the accumulation of large clusters of virus particles and increasing damage to the cell machinery. Eventually the cell may start to destroy itself (by a process called apoptosis) and the virus particles are released and can be carried away in body fluids. If they contact another cell the cycle can be repeated. This process of self-replication continues until the body mobilises its forces to bring it to a halt.

Other viruses have different and more complex lifestyles, but these need not concern us here. Our interest is in those that attack the human airways. Nowadays they can be grouped at the most basic level by the way their genes take over the cells of the host—the 'strategy of the virus genome'. Even amongst this comparatively small group it can be seen that they differ greatly in size and structure.

Class divisions

Viruses used to be classified purely on the basis of the diseases they caused, which depended on what species they could invade and what tissues they

Table 6.1

Family and name	Nucleic acid	Size	Structure	Serotypes	Diseases caused
Picornaviruses					
Rhinoviruses	RNA ss pos	27 nm	Icosahedral	100+	Colds, etc.
Enteroviruses	RNA ss pos	27 nm	Icosahedral	70+	Sore throat, summer flu, meningitis, etc.
Coronaviruses					
Coronaviruses	RNA ss pos	c.120 nm	Helical enveloped	2	Colds
Orthomyxoviruses					
Influenza viruses	RNA ss neg	c.100 nm	Helical enveloped	2 types A or B with strains	Epidemic influenza
Parainfluenza viruses	RNA ss neg	c.220 nm	Helical enveloped	4 parainfluenza	infant colds, pneumonia, etc.
Respiratory syncytical virus (RSV)	RNA ss neg	c.220 nm	Helical enveloped	2	Colds, bronchiolitis
Adenoviruses	DNA ds	c.80 nm	Icosahedral	43	Some cause sore throat, etc.

ss = single stranded; ds = double stranded; neg = negative stranded; pos = positive stranded (see Fig 6.2).
An icosahedral structure gives a rigid shell around the RNA.
Enveloped viruses form particles by 'budding' from the cell surface membrane, which then becomes a flexible envelope. The RNA inside forms a spiral (helix)

damaged. But such categories proved to be insufficiently precise. Our concern is with respiratory disease viruses of humans, which it might be assumed have a number of similarities. However, it transpires that, from a biological point of view, their only common feature is that they are adapted to enter and damage the cells that line the airways of human beings. Otherwise they belong to quite different categories of organisms. Some of their properties are shown in the table.

Chasing the virus

Methods of detecting and studying viruses have developed steadily over the years, fuelled by contributions from laboratories around the world. Although not specifically concerned with respiratory diseases, many of these new ideas have been taken up and adapted to the study of common colds and related conditions. Others have been specifically developed for cold research. Whatever the process of evolution, there has been a dramatic transformation in the methods employed in cold virus research. Four stages can be seen in this process. They are somewhat arbitrary but will help to illustrate the huge advances that have been made by research groups tackling questions such as the spread and treatment of colds.

When cold research began in the 1930s, the only effective method of detecting a cold virus was by inoculating groups of humans in isolation. Influenza viruses could be cultured by inoculating laboratory animals and later embryonated eggs. This period ended in the early 1950s when Enders and others in the USA showed that polioviruses and others could be grown in newly developed tissue cultures. These were made by dispersing human embryo or monkey kidney cells, sticking them to glass on the inside of test tubes, and covering them with a small amount of a simple fluid medium. These cells could be infected by adding virus to the medium; the virus would then grow in the medium and kill the cells. This could be readily observed through the glass of the tube—the so-called cytopathic effect (CPE).

Stage two occurred in the 1950s when specimens from the nose and throat were tested by inoculating tissue cultures. Viruses resembling influenza virus (parainfluenza) were recovered from children in hospital with infections of the airways and pneumonia. Other viruses were grown from tonsil tissue removed by surgeons from adults and children with sore throats, bronchitis, and sometimes pneumonia. These were grouped together as adenoviruses (gland viruses). In 1957, in the USA, two groups using cultures of monkey kidney cells grew a virus (called JH or 2060) from colds in adults, but it was found in only a few cold sufferers. In the late 1950s a method, developed at Salisbury, detected related viruses in the noses of one out of three or four such people—hence rhinoviruses or nose viruses.

The next stage began in 1960 when new laboratory methods were used to discover the basic structure and growth of these new viruses and what diseases they caused. Inoculating volunteers showed that many of the new viruses caused colds, and that antibody against them was present in many people and protected against infection. Children and adults who were falling sick with mild or moderate respiratory illnesses were tested in the US and UK. Most of the new viruses were found in most categories of disease, but rhinoviruses and a further group of viruses, the coronaviruses, could be found in up to 50 percent of common colds. The spread of colds was studied further using specific tests for viruses.

Stage four saw new molecular techniques being used throughout the 1970s and 1980s, making it possible to test for virus proteins. Nucleic acid hybridisation, and later the polymerase chain reaction (PCR), brought limits of detection down to new levels where very small amounts of virus nucleic acid could be detected. In many cases positive readings could be obtained in situations where infectious virus would not have been detected, for instance by inoculating tissue cultures. These methods enabled us to identify virus infections in many more patients. For example, in one study a virus was detected in over 80% children when they had colds.

Tests for immunity

The body has numerous ways of getting rid of foreign substances and so protecting against infection. Cell-mediated immunity is one of these, so called because cells are developed that specifically attack particles and surfaces with foreign proteins and other substances in them. But there is also what is known as humoral, or fluid, immunity. In this system, immune cells produce proteins that float around in the body fluids. These proteins are antibody molecules that are specifically tailored to recognise and combine with certain parts of foreign substances known as antigens. Antibodies and antigens react together very specifically. They can be very useful in the laboratory as well as to the body.

In stage one it was found that antibodies bind to virus particles and make them non-infectious—virus neutralisation. It is then possible to check whether a person has previously been infected with a certain virus by mixing a sample of the virus with some of their blood serum, serum being clotted

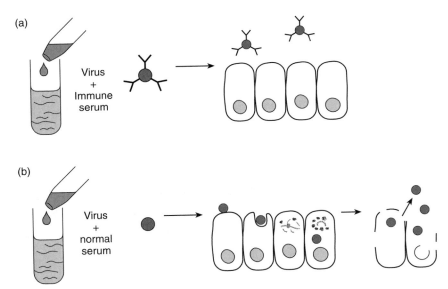

Fig. 6.3 The value of antibodies. (a) Virus neutralisation. A fluid containing virus is added to some immune serum. The latter contains antibodies that combine with specific places on the surface of the virus particle. These prevent the virus from entering and multiplying in cells, which thus remain healthy. (b) By contrast, if virus is added to normal serum, in which there are no antibodies, then the virus is free to infect cells if it reaches them—entering, multiplying, and ultimately killing them. So if cells do *not* degenerate it means that antibody was present.

blood with the red and white cells removed. If the serum neutralises the virus it means the immune system has 'seen' the virus before and made antibodies against it. In a reverse test one could identify or 'type' a new virus by testing it against a serum known to contain specific antibodies.

Since the days of stage two, immunologists have developed many more convenient ways of detecting and measuring antibodies and antigens. In particular antibodies can be combined with fluorescent dyes. If they are placed on infected cells they bind to virus proteins and cannot be washed away. The antibody can then be seen by shining ultraviolet light on the cells and looking for the fluorescent colours of the dye, a process known as immunofluorescence.

Antibodies can also be tagged by attaching radioactive molecules to them and developing 'radioimmunoassays' in which the antibody is detected by measuring the radioactivity that it carries. These reagents can be exquisitely sensitive and specific. Similar tests can be made using antibodies chemically bound to enzymes, known as enzyme-linked immunosorbent assays or ELISA tests.

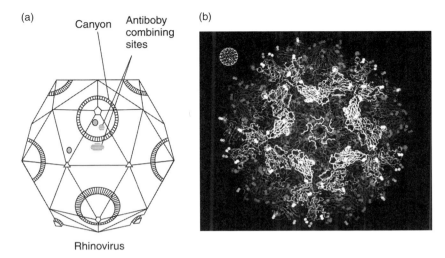

Fig. 6.4 (a) A schematic drawing of a rhinovirus type 14 particle comprising 64 identical triangular facets showing a pole with five-fold symmetry. Round it there is a circular depression (or canyon), and at the bottom of this is an area essential for the particle to enter the cell and release the nucleic acid (RNA) inside it. Four sites of epitopes – areas which stimulate antibody production – are shown and are repeated in similar patterns all over the particle. (b) This computer-generated display (reproduced in colour on the book cover) shows the amino acid strands of the different protiens that make up one side of the rhinovirus particle shell. They form a complex, symmetrical pattern – in this view five identical units are arranged round a central pole. Small parts of the proteins are antigenic – i.e. they stimulate the body to produce specific antibodies. These antigen sites, known as epitopes, are shown as circular dots. (On the cover, the different epitopes are shown in different colours) (Reproduced with permission from D. Stuart)

Useful antibodies can be made by immunising laboratory animals. but there are drawbacks. During stage three, methods were developed for producing 'monoclonal antibodies'. These are made by fusing living, antibody-producing cells with tumour cells. The resulting hybrids grow vigorously and continuously and produce a single type of antibody molecule. The idea was ingenious but many of the practical steps necessary have proved difficult. In spite of this, large numbers of such molecules are now available and can be used for a variety of tasks, ranging from diagnostic tests to purifying difficult molecules.

Work on cell-mediated immunity also suggests further possibilities for studying resistance to infection.

Studying virus interiors

Methods of studying genes and nucleic acids changed out of all recognition in the 1990s. Since then it has become possible to work out the exact

(a)

(b)

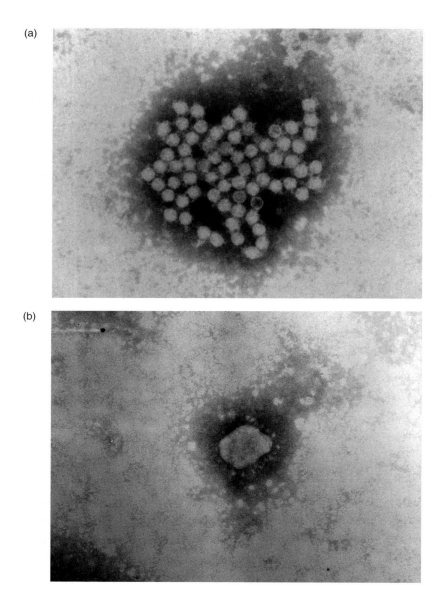

Fig. 6.5 Electron micrograph images of virus particles. These are 'negative contrast' images, so the protein of the viruses appear as light and the surroundings look dark. (a) Particles of rhinovirus type 9 clumped together by antibody. The particles are small and dense and slightly angular in outline. Some are 'empty', where the medium has entered the interior of the particle normally occupied by nucleic acid. (© Barry Dowsett, CAMR.) (b) A particle of coronavirus at the same magnification. Note that it is much larger than a rhinovirus. The outer envelope is curved and flexible and covered with club-shaped projections. These easily detach but also form a halo or crown that gives the virus its name. (From C. R. Madeley.)

nucleotide sequence of the genome, the complete set of genes for all living organisms—animals, plants, and microbes and, most ambitious of all, the tens of thousands of genes embedded in the nucleic acid of every human cell. This was achieved through the Human Genome Project, which used mass-production techniques to work out the basic sequences of the whole of the human genome; and these were published early in 2001. But the first, relatively crude, methods were in use by the late 1970s and could be applied to the nucleic acid of relatively small and simple viruses, such as picornaviruses. Poliovirus was the first to be studied: the virus was purified, and the strands of RNA extracted and converted with enzyme to DNA; this could then be inserted into a bacterium in such a way that the DNA was copied and multiplied. This produced enough of it to permit the use of sequencing methods developed by a Cambridge scientist and Nobel prize-winner, Fred Sanger. The DNA was cut into pieces in a specific way, and the bits spread out in order on a thin membrane, this order indicating the sequence in which they appeared in the strand of DNA. It was then possible to work backwards to the sequence of amino acids that the original RNA specified. This was done in the USA, and then, in the early 1980s in both the USA and the UK, the same approach was used to sequence the genome of rhinovirus type 14.

We at the CCU provided material for the British group under Jeff Almond at Leicester University. There they converted the RNA to DNA and introduced pieces of DNA into bacteria, producing large quantities of the DNA. This was then sequenced. Once they knew the arrangement of the nucleotides they were able to pinpoint that part of the nucleic acid which specified the chain of amino acids making the virus proteins. And, since this was 'written' in the universal triplet code, it told them what the order of amino acids was. In due course rhinovirus 14, which was known to cause colds and grew well in tissue culture, was crystallised and subjected to X-ray crystallography in the USA. This revealed the arrangement in space of the proteins of the outer shell, or capsid, and the amino acids could be placed in position on the capsid. These can now be shown in computer-generated displays (Fig. 6.4).

When we combined virus molecular genetics with the use of monoclonal antibodies we were able to show that antibodies bound to three different chemical patches (epitopes) on the virus when they neutralised it. Most people make these antibodies and they all produce immunity. The clever virus can change these patches so they resist antibodies, but the even cleverer body shoots at up to three different patches at once, and that is more than the virus can cope with. The body wins.

It seemed to us that we could use the DNA prepared in bacteria to study our rhinoviruses and detect them in patients. A study of the sequence showed that the information for making proteins was situated in the middle of the RNA strand. The beginning of the strand did not code for proteins but might relate to some function that was important for all rhinoviruses. It was an area we needed to study, and for this we needed more DNA—and someone who could give plenty of time to the project.

At about this time an enthusiastic visiting scientist from Kuwait, Widad al-Nakib, arrived at the unit. He had already done important work on antiviral drugs and was now keen to have a go at this project. He and I drove first to Leicester to get the advice of the team there on how best to make probes and run tests. Armed with this information and some bacteria that would make DNA copies of this part of the genome for us, Widad then set out to find a way to detect rhinovirus nucleic acid in culture fluids and nasal fluids from volunteers. It was to prove a difficult task: the search went on for several years and was still in progress after he had left.

Chain reaction does the trick

The first method we tried was to extract RNA, which could be tricky, and put it on a plastic membrane. Copy-DNA, grown from the bacteria, was 'labelled' with radioactive phosphorus and purified. A solution of this was laid over the membrane and then washed off. If the DNA sequence matched part of the RNA they bonded together (hybridised), and so the DNA and the radioactive phosphorus became stuck to the membrane. This could not be observed using any optical system: the answer lay in another part of the spectrum. X-ray film was laid on the membrane in the dark, and after several days was taken off and developed. If DNA had bound, a blackened area appeared where the RNA had been put on the membrane. This method detected RNA from many different serotypes of rhinovirus grown in laboratory cultures and in the nasal washing from some of our volunteers with rhinovirus colds (Fig. 6.6).

Methods have much improved since then, using a process which magnifies the 'target' on the RNA to the point where it can be recognised visually in some cases. This is the PCR mentioned earlier, which involves the use of enzymes and short lengths of synthetic DNA (oligonucleotide primers) to direct a polymerase enzyme to a particular stretch of nucleic acid (the 'target'), resulting in a million-fold increase in material. The exact identity of the material can still be checked using hybridisation, which makes the test very specific as well as sensitive.

Such methods are now used widely to detect and measure amounts of virus nucleic acid in the blood of patients with AIDS, infectious jaundice,

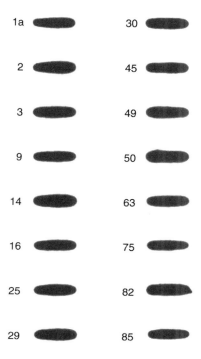

Fig. 6.6 A molecular method for detecting rhinovirus nucleic acid. The RNA from 16 different serotypes of rhinovirus has been placed on a membrane. This was washed and then exposed to a nucleic acid probe that binds to a sequence found on all types of rhinoviruses but not on other picornaviruses. The membrane was washed again and laid on X-ray film in the dark. The probe was radio-labelled so the developed film showed blackening where the probe had been bound to the membrane. The figure shows that all the types of virus were detected.

and other diseases. They are not generally used to study colds. However, a medical researcher, Sebastian Johnston from Southampton University, our local medical school, having learned the methods at CCU, developed them further and used them to study colds in patients with asthma. Working with a group of children in the area he and his colleagues showed that a range of viruses caused colds which then went on to trigger attacks of wheezing. And usually rhinovirus nucleic acid was found in the nose, and this was confirmed by growing the virus in tissue culture.

This example shows how an interest in the ultimate details of a virus can provide methods with which to explore the causes of other illnesses and not just of colds. But we need more than this insight, based on science, to help us understand what is going on in an 'ordinary' common cold. We

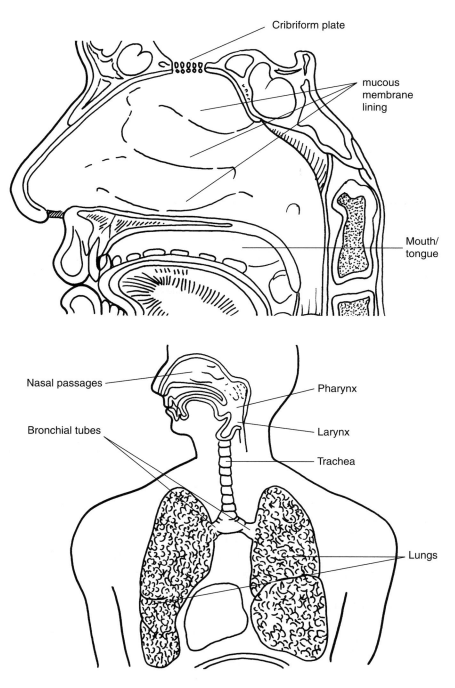

Fig. 6.7 The human nose and airways, whose functions are summarised in the text.

need to study those parts of the body which come under attack from cold viruses.

Take a deep breath

Our ability to breathe is something we take for granted. And that is because we have an apparatus for the purpose so remarkable that we are usually unaware of what it is doing. I remember medical students being asked to listen to a patient talking about his difficult breathing so they could appreciate their own good fortune and recognise that this facility was not shared by everyone. We only take notice of our upper airways when they start to misbehave—usually when we catch a cold. But do we ever wonder how the nose is constructed and how it actually works?

It starts at the two nostrils. Behind them are two quite narrow slits, the nasal passages. In some animal species these have a complex shape, but in us they are relatively simple. On the inner side is a smooth flat surface while, on the outer, three curled ridges stick out. And there are small openings which lead into air cavities or sinuses which are, so to speak, excavated out of the bones of the face and forehead. The back of the nose leads into the throat or pharynx which is a dual purpose passageway. Food and drink enter at the front of the mouth, pass through to the back, and then descend down the gullet or oesophagus. Air enters through the nose or mouth and goes past the back of the tongue, through the voice box, or larynx, and into the windpipe, or trachea. This carries it down the smaller tubes, bronchi and bronchioles, into the air cells. On the return journey, the air flows out through the nose or mouth. Two valve mechanisms help to control these movements. One is the soft palate with the little uvula hanging from it—readily seen in a mirror. This lifts when food is going down and prevents it going up into the nose. The other, the epiglottis, which is behind the tongue, tilts backwards and downwards to prevent food going into the voice box. The nervous system helps, too, because it automatically stops us breathing when we swallow. It also pushes us to close our mouths when we want to chew or swallow. So an infant or child with a blocked nose can have difficulty sucking or eating.

Some defences

Our airways are lined with a remarkable tissue, the mucous membrane, which extends from the nose down to the smallest bronchiole. This has two kinds of cells along its surface. The first of these, with the help of small mucus glands, secrete a layer of sticky mucus onto the surface. The second are referred to as 'ciliated' because their surface consists of tiny hair-like processes that beat vigorously and systematically in the mucus layer. Like an escalator or ripples on the surface of a pond, these move the mucus up the bronchi until it reaches the throat and is swallowed. When we reach the nose this movement of the mucus, now moving backwards into the throat, still continues for the most part, but there is also a small forward movement from the very front of the nose.

Only occasionally do we notice this wonderfully efficient, air-conditioning system at work. Air always contains dust particles. The larger ones stick to the mucus in the nose and the smaller ones are caught in the lower airways. Spend

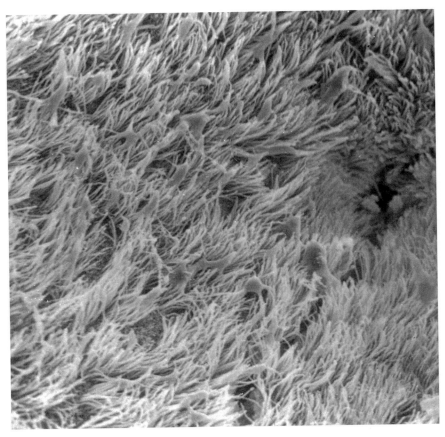

Fig. 6.8 The lining membrane of the airways as seen by the scanning electron microscope. It is covered by fine hair-like projections (cilia) that beat constantly and systematically and drive along the mucus that lies over them. The mucus comes from glandular cells between the cilia and from small mucus glands which open out here and there onto the surface. (From the collection of S. E. Reed.)

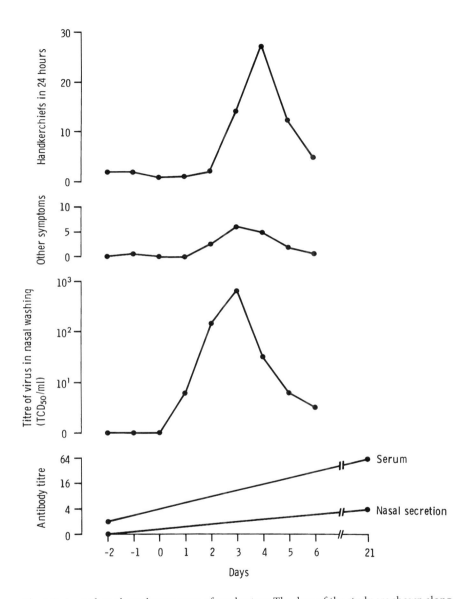

Fig. 6.9 A graph to show the response of a volunteer. The days of the study are shown along the bottom and the various measurements made are plotted vertically. After the quarantine period virus is given on day zero. At first there is no response but then the nose begins to run (top panel) and virus is found in the nose. In a few days these return to normal, but tests on blood and nose secretions show that the body has made antibodies against the virus. These will persist for a long time and prevent infection if the same virus type is given again.

time in a dusty place and we soon notice dried black mucus in the nostrils or we may clear our throats and find black mucus on a handkerchief. The mechanism is sometimes helped when a particularly irritating particle or chemical triggers the mucus glands to produce extra mucus. The net result is that the particles are not allowed to penetrate too far. The system has done its job.

The mucous membrane also warms and humidifies the air. Water evaporates from the warm mucus and gradually heats the air so that it reaches the air cells at body temperature. It is easy to feel the warmth with a hand as the air is breathed out again; the water can be detected by breathing on a cold mirror.

The 'mucus escalator' also defends the body against bacteria and viruses that are inhaled riding on dust particles. Another form of defence is provided by clusters of special cells of the immune system which surround the throat, forming the tonsils and adenoids. These can take up bacteria and viruses and launch an immune counterattack.

These systems are not always enough. But there are other mechanisms that can come into play when needed. These are triggered whenever something very important needs to be done, like stopping bleeding or maintaining breathing. In the case of colds there are nerve endings in the mucous membrane that detect when there is an excess of mucus or a very irritant particle. These produce nerve impulses which travel up to nerve centres in the spinal cord and the base of the brain. There they trigger an automatic, organised response. If the message comes from the lower airways, muscles in the chest and abdomen contract, and the larynx closes and then opens suddenly. Compressed air is suddenly released and moves up and out through the mouth at very high speed; so fast in fact that large particles and small collections of mucus are picked up and blown out of the body—in a cough. A similar reflex blows unwanted material out of the nose—in a sneeze.

These examples illustrate how adept the body is in bringing its general purpose mechanisms into play to deal with a particular attack or type of damage. They also show how the symptoms and signs of particular diseases are often due to the body mobilising its forces in this way. The conclusion is somewhat reassuring: viruses may be very clever but only rarely do they come out on top.

Fortunately nearly all colds are mild, and the symptoms (what we feel) and signs (what can be seen or measured) reflect the way the body is successfully counterattacking against the virus invasion. All cold viruses produce rather similar colds though they do vary from person to person. A typical illness might start with some irritation and soreness at the back of the nose and throat. Then the nose feels uncomfortable, partly blocked and begins to run. Sometimes there is sneezing and the discharge from the nose changes from clear (mucoid) to partly cloudy (mucopurulent). There may be a headache at first and the patient may feel unwell generally, but this soon passes and the main problem is with the blocked or running nose. After two or three days the nose begins to feel better but there may be a cough, often linked with the feeling that mucus is running down the throat. Sometimes the blocked nose or the cough make it difficult to sleep. Within about a week most of the symptoms have gone or are substantially better. If the illness is mainly focused in the throat it is still most likely to be due to a virus, but about one in ten such cases are due to a bacterium (streptococcal sore throat).

Anatomy of a cold

Let us imagine we can put ourselves under a powerful microscope and see in detail the remarkable sequence of events which occurs when we are exposed to one of the viruses of a very ordinary cold. When someone with such a cold sneezes in our direction we may expect to catch it. But quite often we do not. There are two possible reasons: either the virus does not reach us or it is a virus we have had before. If the latter then we will be carrying the antibodies that will wipe it out. Some will be in the mucus where the virus lands. It may get past this and kill a few cells, but these cells can call up other antibodies in the blood and these can snuff out the beginnings of the infection. The job will be done discreetly and we will not know it is happening.

Whatever the situation there is no way of telling at this stage whether we have been smitten or not. If a virus, let us assume it is a rhinovirus, does get through it will land on the mucous membrane of the nose, get moved along by the cilia, and quickly attach itself to a cell. Absorbed by the cell it immediately begins to multiply and within hours the infected cell breaks open and large numbers of new virus particles come out and spread to surrounding cells. We continue to feel well and stay well for about two days, though in the second day virus particles may be found in the nose. The first phase of an attack is always like this.

The next stage is when we start to feel discomfort. The body's emergency communication system goes into action, with cells invaded by viruses releasing what are known as chemical messengers. These are specialised molecules that attach to specific spots on the surfaces of cells and make them respond as instructed, in a variety of ways. They form a complicated network affecting many types of cells and are classified into a number of different groups bearing names such as cytokines, lymphokines, and interleukins (IL6 is an example of this last group). Some of these are being exploited in treatments designed either to increase or decrease their effects in diseases–for example, in the use of drugs to block the tumour necrosis factor alpha (TNFα) in rheumatoid arthritis.

The messengers make blood vessels dilate, and attract white blood cells; and antibodies leak from the blood into the membrane of the nose. Antibodies may combine with virus proteins, and the combined particles bind to other blood proteins and trigger more chemical messengers. Damaged cells can release messengers that stir the nerve endings at the back of the nose and top of the throat, and these may induce a feeling of soreness. They also trigger the reflexes that make the nose run and cause us to sneeze. This helps us by clearing the nose, but it may also help the virus to find another home.

These infections have effects outside the nose. The passages to the sinuses and middle ear are often blocked so that fluids build up and the pressure inside them is no longer adjusted. These pressure changes may cause pain, for example in the cheeks, forehead, and ear, and can be unpleasant when driving up or down a hill, or when a plane is taking off or landing. The chemical messengers can also be absorbed into the circulation and carried to the nervous system. At the base of the brain they may signal the body's thermostat mechanism to raise the temperature, resulting in our feeling chilly and even shivering. Headache, muscle ache, tiredness, and a feeling of illness may result.

Viruses can spread to the ear and sinuses but are more likely to cause trouble by going down into the lower airways, producing the same sort of effect as in the nose. If the bronchi are irritated there may be a 'dry' cough, though if they also secrete too much fluid there will be a 'moist ' cough and clear sputum will come up to be swallowed or spat out.

A cough can be triggered by mucus running down the back of the throat and can continue for a week or two even if the rest of the cold has cleared up. The membrane takes time to grow new cells to replace the damaged ones, and during that time some inflammation and extra mucus may remain to trigger the cough reflex.

Most symptoms will usually be gone or much improved after five days or so, but sometimes the cough and pain or general symptoms get worse. The discharge becomes yellow or green and this may well mean that bacteria have multiplied on the damaged membrane, causing more serious harm to the tissues and releasing their own poisons into the circulation.

Whether there are complications or not, the body usually produces antibodies against the virus that persist in the blood for years and in the nose for a shorter time. These will neutralise any virus of the same type if breathed in again. The trouble is that there are a great many viruses with different antigens on their surfaces, which therefore need different antibodies to neutralise them. As there are so many, over 100 rhinoviruses, for example, and more than 200 cold viruses in total, it is not surprising that we often seem to have no immunity to colds. We must be grateful that there are not a similar number of measles viruses, for it would be impossible to produce a vaccine that would cope with them all; and we would be liable to a hundred attacks of measles before we were totally immune.

Some complications

Virus may be inhaled into the lower airways and infect them, causing bronchitis, although a cough during a cold may be due to irritation in the throat.

Virus may spread to the middle ear, along the Eustachian tube. Infection there can cause mucus to accumulate, and if bacteria get in as well there can be a serious middle ear infection (*otitis media*). This happens more readily in babies and small children.

The virus can quite easily travel from the nose to the air sinuses, and recent evidence shows that even in mild colds mucus builds up in the sinuses and is cleared away by the cilia as the cold subsides. But, once again, if bacteria get in they may set up a more serious inflammation, bacterial sinusitis, and this can happen in both young and old.

Certain viruses tend to damage particular parts of the lower airways. For example, parainfluenza viruses attack the larynx and respiratory syncytial virus the bronchioles of infants. So croup, laryngitis, or bronchiolitis may follow if they infect.

People with long-term problems involving the airways—for example those with asthma, bronchitis, and emphysema or heart failure—may get worse after a cold and this also applies to patients with diabetes or kidney disease.

Finally, there is the possibility that the illness is not a cold but influenza. One clue is that influenza tends to have less effect on the nose while producing more severe general symptoms such as aches, shivering, and a higher temperature, and many sufferers want to take to their beds. But this is 'clinical' influenza which can occasionally be caused by any of a number of different viruses. The 'real' influenza viruses, types A and B, come in winter epidemics and are the usual cause of this illness. It is becoming more important to recognise these because they are serious and can kill. There are vaccines against them, and new and better drug treatments are being developed.

Coping with colds

The medical profession has become increasingly involved at the point of birth and of death but, in between those two significant milestones, it still remains helpless when faced with the common cold—well illustrated by an old joke. Doctor tells patient: 'You've got a nasty cold, but I've got nothing to cure it. Give me a call if it turns into pneumonia—I could definitely treat that.' Researchers may see the common cold as an interesting biological event but for most people it is an unpleasant experience which they want to bring to an end as quickly as possible. This usually means waiting patiently at home for the whole thing to go away.

Modern science has changed the way medicine is practised in so many fields but has failed to produce any radically new treatments for the common cold. It is true that our understanding of colds has grown immensely and should help us to deal with them in a more rational way. But old habits die hard, and any new knowledge which has emerged has been absorbed into a large and miscellaneous collection of ideas about the condition. Just as Catholic beliefs have been superimposed on pagan traditions in South America and elsewhere, so scientific facts on the cause of colds are entertained alongside apparently incompatible folklore.

A mother may know that colds are caused by viruses but, in her heart, she still believes the illness is due to being chilled in a cold wind, a draught, or getting caught in the rain. So she will send her children to change their wet socks with the warning 'if you don't want to come down with a cold'. Her attitude is conditioned by her own experience as a child when she received similar instructions from her parents. Similarly, someone may know that there are no effective treatments for the viruses that cause colds but still recommend a particular hot toddy to cure the condition, 'because it works for me'.

At least we are now spared the worst excesses of the patent medicine culture in which outrageous claims were made for useless coloured liquids. Official action has put paid to that, and most practitioners would not now prescribe a linctus as a cold cure. Nevertheless, it is still possible to buy an over-the-counter mixture to relieve cold symptoms. These are formulated on a fairly sound therapeutic basis but they still cost significantly more than simpler home remedies or the same drugs bought as generic preparations.

In the Far East and many developing countries there are numerous complementary medical systems offering treatment. Indeed WHO often encourages cold sufferers to use these traditional, alternative, or complementary methods, and it is becoming easier in Western countries to find practitioners who offer these treatments. There is often little or no evidence that they actually improve the course of a cold but they are usually cheap and may not have the adverse effects of normal Western medicines. Furthermore, if the practitioner involved knows how to recognise the early stages of a serious condition he will refer such a patient on. Meanwhile the mildly ill patient benefits from the extra personal attention and concern.

This seems to me to be good, practical therapy because if patients push too hard for attention the result may be a prescription for a potentially harmful antibiotic to send them on their way. Even alternative therapies have their dangers: some herbal infusions or 'bush teas' can be toxic. And acupuncture, which provides objective benefit in some health problems, must be performed with proper sterile techniques, or serious infection, such as the hepatitis B virus, can result.

All this illustrates the old medical saying 'If there are ten different treatments for a condition then none of them is any good.' A bit unfair, perhaps, since we shall see that simple symptomatic treatment can make people feel significantly better while their body is curing the disease. But it is not a satisfactory state of affairs. We should inform people better on the nature of colds and the best ways of managing them, and press on and try and develop an economical and effective way of preventing or treating them.

Things have improved, however. Instead of a lone GP with access to a few effective treatments we have group practices with nurses and other ancillary professionals. If they don't treat conditions themselves they are the gateway to wide-ranging and effective specialist services. But acute respiratory infections are not seen as a real health problem.

Treating the symptoms

There are no drugs that will directly attack the cold viruses. We can only deal with the results they produce. But treating the symptoms will at least make us 'feel better while we're getting better', to paraphrase Dr Andrewes. People vary a good deal in what they dislike and what they find helpful, but there are some good general principles to follow, starting with one from the ancient physicians 'primum non nocere': firstly do not harm.

All medicines have some undesirable side effects so we should treat only the symptoms that bother us, forgetting those we can readily tolerate and, particularly, those we do not have. This usually means using single medicines and not mixtures sold as cold cures. If a sore throat or headache is the problem use aspirin or ibuprofen—both members of the non-steroidal anti-inflammatory drug family. But a hot, sweet drink can also do the job.

Mixtures may contain drugs to constrict blood vessels and so reduce the blockage in the nose. If taken by mouth these will affect blood vessels throughout the body and could be harmful to people with high blood pressure. Drops or inhalations can be employed to treat just the blood vessels in the nose but, used frequently, they may make the membranes swell rather than helping them to shrink.

Antihistamine drugs have become popular in the treatment of colds even though histamine plays no part in the development of a cold. It follows that they will not provide a cure. Their value to the cold sufferer is in providing a degree of sedation as an aid to sleep and in blocking certain nerve endings (anticholinergic action), as a means of drying up nasal secretion. But a traditional remedy, such as a hot bath and a drink, may be just as effective, easing the nose and helping towards a good night's sleep. The nose dries up a good deal in sleep anyway, and next morning usually feels a better day. Some people find a steam kettle in the room helpful, especially if the air is dry.

A persistent cough can be controlled with compounds related to codeine, such as folcodeine. But this is best avoided if the cough is not too irritating, and particularly if it is doing a useful job by raising mucus.

Buying drugs sold under their generic names rather than the more expensive trade names will save money. Knowing about dosage and possible side effects is important, as is ensuring that they do not add to the dosage of any other drug being taken.

Antibiotics have become such powerful allies in the fight against infections that they have acquired a reputation as cure-alls. And so let it be said right now that much painstaking research has shown that *antibiotics are of no benefit in colds*. But patients ask for them and doctors offer them just to show that they care and want to help. The trouble is, they all cause harmful effects in a proportion of patients. Furthermore, antibiotics are now becoming less effective in treating serious infections precisely because their frequent use for colds has brought an increase in drug-resistant bacteria in the community. Every time a bacterium survives drug treatment it joins the growing ranks of those that cannot be killed by certain groups of antibiotics. As far as bacteria are concerned familiarity breeds contempt.

Other treatments and preventatives

The most effective way of avoiding colds is to live in complete isolation from the rest of the human race. Other people are the problem. But the majority of us, for whom such advice may seem a touch impractical, must look for more workable alternatives. There are many of these, although quite a number are of doubtful value.

Using medicated nasal tissues has been suggested, on limited scientific evidence. Good hand hygiene helps to avoid many infections but does little, if anything, to prevent colds in average circumstances.

We know from our research that children with colds are good at spreading them and that people with chronic illnesses are liable to complications if they catch them. Keeping the two apart in the home is a sensible precaution, at least during the first day or two when the risk of infection is at its greatest.

Many still believe in taking large and regular doses of vitamin C (ascorbic acid) to ward off colds. Our research showed no significant benefit, and this was confirmed in many other trials. But some scientists believe that such treatment has a small positive effect. My own view is that the money is better spent on a good quality mixed diet which will benefit all aspects of health.

At one time it was customary to remove tonsils and adenoids to prevent childhood respiratory diseases. If they are chronically infected or obstructing the airways the operation can be valuable, but there is good evidence that it does not prevent colds. Many unnecessary operations must have been performed for this reason.

Strongly smelling substances, such as menthol, oil of eucalyptus, or friars balsam have always been popular in the treatment of colds. They may help the airways when inhaled in steam, but the benefit could be due to the steam as much as the odour. In fact a study of the effect of menthol on the physiology of the nose showed that it removed the blocked sensation although measurement demonstrated that the airway was not opened up.

Various alternative medicines have been proposed but none, to our knowledge, have been assessed by a properly controlled clinical trial. In the People's Republic of China patients can opt to be treated by either Western or traditional medicine, and we gather that both are used. Acupuncture seems to be popular, using a site at the base of the thumb. Other practitioners use moxibustion—where a soft wool (moxa) produced from certain dried leaves is burnt close to the skin—but we have not been able to find any reports of clinical evaluation trials.

Striking a balance

All this suggests that, as far as colds are concerned, we should be aware of our symptoms but not overreact to them. They may make us feel uncomfortable but they are also a sign that the body is getting to grips with the problem. Nevertheless we must take note of what our bodies are telling us. For primary health care to work well, people need to distinguish between a minor health problem that will recover on its own and one that needs medical attention. For example, vomiting, high fever, shortage of breath, coughing blood, or a lack of improvement within, say, five days would be clear evidence of something more serious which might not be a cold at all.

In recent years we have learned a great deal about the details of what can happen in cells, blood vessels, and the nervous and immune systems, both in the laboratory and in people with colds. However, only the broad outlines and the general principles are clear and generally agreed. Current ideas are likely to be modified in time because this area of science is changing rapidly.

CHAPTER 7

Oh to be a volunteer

The founding of the CCU somehow caught the public imagination. And this, of course, was because of the volunteers. There was nothing like it, or them, anywhere else in the world. When the Crown Film Unit produced a series of wartime films entitled *Britain can make it*, one of the last of these featured the CCU. It began with a woman sneezing at a conveyer belt in an armaments factory and ended with cheerful volunteers in their rooms, and a scientist handling vials of possible virus.

After the success of the initial volunteer programme, trials for up to 30 volunteers were organised throughout the year, generally running from Tuesday of one week to Friday of the next. Easter and bank holidays were usually included but the unit closed over Christmas. A very large number would be needed throughout the course of the year, and it was soon realised that students could not fill all the available places. The general public would have to be involved. But how to approach them? And how would they react to the idea of being guinea pigs in this new research project? They might think they would be given terrible colds and have to take to their beds; undergo painful tests and treatment; or be placed in solitary confinement. Our publicity claimed that it would be more like a country holiday, but would they believe us?

Such concern proved to be groundless—the public didn't mind at all, quite the contrary. But ways had still to be found to get the message across.

What the papers say

When I was a trainee at Sheffield Medical School in the 1940s I was given quite clear guidance on how to regard the press. It was alright for the local papers to report official events at the university. It was not alright for me to talk about research in progress. This must be reported, when completed, to an audience of clinical scientists. Anyway, we were told, if you did try talking to the press the journalists would simply get it all wrong.

There was a more open attitude in the USA when I was there in the 1950s. Newspapers such as the *New York Times* were publishing major and well-informed articles on medical science. Such subjects were clearly seen to be of general interest, in contrast with the attitude in Britain. However, my ivory tower research department was an unlikely candidate for press curiosity, and nobody came to interview me. But I do remember a few enquiries after I had given a paper.

Major developments and epidemics, of course, have always received wide press coverage. We know that Pasteur in the nineteenth century staged public shows to demonstrate the effect of his vaccines with the intention that they should be widely reported. Influenza also attracts plenty of column inches because of the high mortality and social disruption it has frequently caused. But I know of no similar publicity in connection with the investigation of colds. Medical journals, of course, reported on cold research when the subject was discussed at medical society meetings, but this was all relatively low key—certainly not something likely to reach the ear of the general public. If we were to get volunteers in the numbers we required then we had to change our attitude. We needed publicity.

The MRC did not give us an advertising budget, so the unit usually sent out press releases, which reported on some interesting discovery that was considered sufficient to excite interest and concluded with the comment that more volunteers would be needed if the research was to continue. Something was usually said about the trial procedures, the pleasant conditions, and what a good holiday it could be. Press conferences were also quite common, enabling journalists to see who the scientists were and ask questions. Since it was not customary for research workers to talk publicly about their work, it came as quite a surprise to new members of staff to discover that this was part of their job at the CCU.

Our work, as a result, was reported from time to time and our need for volunteers would also be mentioned, often under rather frivolous headlines such as 'Not to be sneezed at'. Occasional pieces on radio and television were responsible for making it more generally known that there are around 200 viruses causing colds rather than the single one that most people had imagined up until then. And people might then understand that this is probably why we have so many colds.

Without nationwide media courage we would almost certainly not have had enough offers of help to keep the volunteer programme going for so many years. Of course the publicity was only effective because it met with a positive response in a small but motivated fraction of the population. But by seeking publicity we also risked compromise. Most journalists grasped perfectly well the way we described our scientific results. We used simple

FREE 10 DAY AUTUMN AND WINTER BREAK

YOU MAY NOT WIN A NOBEL PRIZE BUT

YOU COULD HELP FIND A CURE FOR THE COMMON COLD

400 people come every year aged 18–50
Many return annually
Warm and comfortable accommodation with single bedded rooms
Travel expenses paid south of Edinburgh
£1.25 per day pocket money
Excellent opportunity to study, walks or just relaxing,
Write:

**COMMON COLD UNIT, SALISBURY, WILTS. SP2 88W.
Tel: 0722-22485**

between 9 a.m. and 5 p.m.

Fig. 7.1 A typical low-key advertisement for volunteers.

language but kept the sense intact and honest. But we knew that things we had not said were likely to appear between quotation marks, and that there might well be headlines that neither we nor the journalists could alter. It was easy to let slip a phrase which suggested that a useful treatment might emerge soon, whereas what we meant was that we had some hopeful new results which were not yet ready to apply. But our need for volunteers was often mentioned at the end of the article and this was what mattered most.

Perfect for pairs

Journalists sometimes came to visit the unit when trials were on, and one or two came as volunteers. One pretended she was a teacher but her cover was blown when she received a phone call from her editor during the trial. She left before it ended.

Perhaps the most memorable interchange in a conference was when Christopher Andrewes made what he later described as a grave error. These are his words.

> I explained that we wanted our volunteers for ten days at a time, twenty-four every fortnight, and that, as solitary confinement would be dull, we would house them in pairs—friends or married couples. On the spur of the moment I added, it would do nicely for honeymooners. How the reporters scribbled that down, and we have never been allowed to forget it! Though we have only had a very few honeymoon couples in seventeen years, the hospital is still known to many as the place where the honeymooners go.

In fact the result was almost entirely beneficial. Apart from some extra work and a certain amount of embarrassment it provided a lot of free publicity, and we certainly needed that. It also meant that some people found it difficult to take the place seriously, and indeed it featured in at least one novel: Iris Murdoch's *Under the Net*. In this, a man called Jake says

> It was through the common cold that I first met Hugo. This was in a period when I was particularly short of cash, and things went very ill indeed with me until I discovered an incredibly charitable arrangement whereby I could get free board and lodging in exchange for being a guinea pig in a cold cure experiment...at a delightful country house.

The CCU had become widely known from the 1950s onwards, and people would say how frequently they kept on hearing about it. Magazine editors and programme makers would contact us for help if they were planning an item on colds. When Thames Television approached the medical superintendent he supplied them with the information they wanted but included a paragraph stressing that we were always short of volunteers and how necessary they were for our work. Hundreds of letters and phone calls would follow a press event, a broadcast, or a magazine article, but only a small proportion of these would lead to a volunteer coming. Our best ambassadors were the volunteers themselves. They would tell their friends how much they had enjoyed the experience, and some of these would pluck up courage and try it for themselves.

We were able to run these trials so regularly because British people were extraordinarily willing to cooperate in this way. Some did it as a way of contributing to society, like being a blood donor. Others were saying thank you to the medical world for something it had done to treat a relative or friend. Others came for a cheap, quiet holiday or rest, the best way they knew to escape from a stressful job. And most would admit that they liked the idea of cooperating with a research team to discover something about the cause and treatment of a troublesome group of diseases. They were always interested in the work that was going on and would want to know whether they had been given active virus or dummy, drug or placebo. And they were often pleased to know that they would appear as a dot on a graph or a digit when the paper was published in *The Lancet*.

Visitors from Germany, France, or the USA said they could never get such a system to work in their countries and with their citizens—particularly since our people were not paid anything. In spite of this nearly 20 000 volunteers took part in these trials during the lifetime of the CCU.

Life as a volunteer

The unit changed in superficial ways over the years but the main patterns of its life and impact on volunteers remained the same. This was surprising in view of the huge changes in society between 1946 and 1990 but, in this little corner of Wiltshire, time moved slowly. Such calm progress through so many decades is surely a tribute to the good judgement of those who set it up.

A typical volunteer would hear about the unit through a magazine or television news item. More than one man admitted, rather sheepishly, that it was

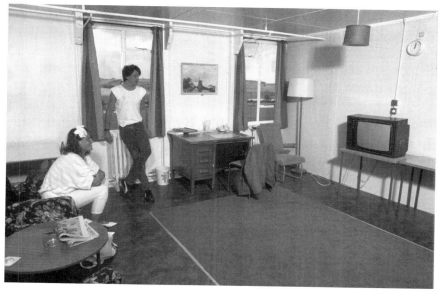

Fig. 7.2 The sitting room in a flat.

by listening to 'Woman's Hour' on the radio! A postcard notice displayed at the Town Hall in Dover was sufficient to attract one volunteer, the only person known to have been enticed by this method. He later wrote to us about his, not wholly enjoyable, experiences:

> Dr Hall (the medical superintendent at the time) was a kindly, avuncular man and Matron Bailey…rather brisk. I do remember that I was given the father and mother of all colds. I was on a drugs trial and six times a day I had to squirt some concoction up my nose from a plastic container. Each time I felt my nose had been blasted off. Towards the end of the trial Matron began to feel sorry for me and gave me a medicine, which was awful.

The man also wrote to find out what he had been given, to be told that he received rhinoviruses 9 and 31. The summary report on his condition was: score 49, mild reaction. 'MILD!', he exclaimed, 'what on earth do you call a strong reaction?' In fact the reaction term referred to whether he had temperature or other flu-like symptoms and was not supposed to indicate the intensity of his feelings. In spite of this the CCU worked its unique magic and he came nine more times. On one occasion he developed a romantic feeling for a woman volunteer, an oboist who played with a London orchestra. 'I had brought my guitar down with me', he said, 'and we played duets at 30 feet while the trial lasted, and closer at the end.'

Students saw it as a cheap holiday, with uninterrupted writing and study time, and the opportunity for some splendid country walks. Inviting a friend to come along would then ensure agreeable company. People enjoyed the experience, as was shown by the fact that the largest number came through the influence of some previous volunteer.

Another woman, a newsagent who wanted time to study, had four or five colds in 14 visits and enjoyed the restful atmosphere. Except, perhaps, for the time when a deckchair collapsed and trapped her finger in the framework. Her screams for help nearly caused a couple of volunteers to break the isolation rules but, fortunately, medical help arrived quickly and resolved their dilemma. The woman's finger was soon made well again and she responded with considerable gratitude calling the staff 'the kindest, nicest bunch of people one could ever hope to meet…to name a few would be an injustice to the rest'. But she did mention the ex-mayor of Salisbury who was 'calling on us daily for nose drippings'. But that's another story.

When potential volunteers rang the unit they would be greeted by a pleasant voice with a promise to send some details and an application form. The information would explain why trials were needed and what questions were being tackled at the time. There would be a description of the facilities and what happened in a trial, plus a list of dates of trials for which there were still vacancies. The booking form was rather like that for a travel agent arranging a holiday—apart from a few extra details and no mention of any charges.

Applicants would receive a reply to say they were accepted, followed by a travel warrant. This could then be converted to a ticket at their local railway station. When the trial date arrived they would take a train, on a Monday or a Tuesday, with a bag packed for a short country holiday in Salisbury. They would see the cathedral spire from the carriage window as they stepped onto the platform and might well notice one or two other passengers looking around uncertainly. Outside would be a man with a welcoming smile and a minibus who seemed to know who they were. He would then whisk them off through the old streets of Salisbury to the southern outskirts, onto the Blandford Road and, after a short distance, through some white timber gates and onto an open grassy site.

Almost inevitably their hearts must have sunk a little as they viewed for the first time the rows of dull green huts. Their first stop would be at one of these, identified by a rather faded notice announcing 'Office' at one end. Once inside they were welcomed by the office staff and told the number of the flat to which they had been assigned. From there they were led along wooden walkways and shown round their rooms. It says much for the general air of friendliness and the comfort of the accommodation that the initial impressions and any possible misgivings seemed to evaporate very quickly.

The flats were certainly comfortable, if a little basic by today's standards. Each was constructed on a similar pattern. The door opened onto a narrow corridor, the floor covered in brown linoleum with walls and ceiling painted cream or a light green. This led first to a spacious sitting room with easy chairs, some small tables, a radio or television set, and a dart board. On one table were maps of the unit and the surrounding area with suggested walks, a note of the games available in the recreation huts, and a list of books in the unit library. There was also a note of board games to be borrowed and a form on which to write a shopping list of all the things that the volunteer had inevitably forgotten to bring. These would be bought in the town and delivered next day.

Further doors opened onto single bedrooms, two in some flats and three in others, each furnished with an inner-sprung American bed, a pine chest, and a wardrobe cupboard. Beyond the bedrooms was a medical room with a table, chairs, and a bed to serve as a couch for inoculating and so on. Next to that was a small kitchen with cupboard and drawers for cutlery, crockery, and

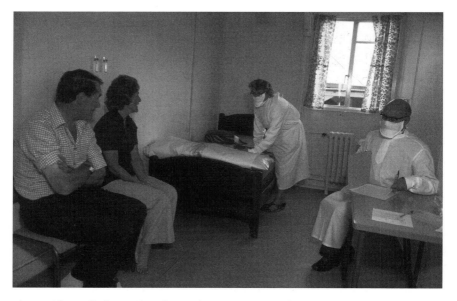

Fig. 7.3 The medical superintendent and matron visiting a flat for the daily examination. The bed was used when inoculating the volunteers.

stores. Also in this room were a table and chairs where volunteers would normally eat their meals. At the end of the corridor was a bathroom or shower room and toilet. And behind these, out of sight, was a compartment for the oil-fired boiler which provided domestic hot water and heated the solid, cast iron radiators that stood under most of the windows.

We might think the conditions austere but, in the first years of peace, volunteers felt quite cosseted. A journalist visited the unit in 1947 and 'found the volunteers isolated in pairs, living in very comfortable flats, with meals supplied, bathrooms fitted with showers, central heating and every possible comfort.' She then added, 'I was impressed by the friendliness of the staff and the general cleanliness of the place. It looked so cared for, and I was amazed that wartime huts could be so spacious and warm.' Some volunteers travelled down from as far away as Scotland; and so the flats represented something of a haven after such a journey. One visitor, used to Scottish tenements, felt that 'bungalows' or 'terraced cabins' would be more appropriate descriptions.

Adjusting to the rules

After settling-in volunteers would walk across to the dining room. This took up almost half a hut and had a huge heated counter left by the Americans. The volunteers were seated at a couple of long tables with some members of the staff and served with a hot meal, usually roast meat and vegetables and a homely pudding. They then moved to the far end of the room and found themselves a seat for coffee, often in one or other of the huge armchairs that also came with the building. Coffee time merged into a series of short talks explaining what was to happen and the strict isolation rules: don't go into shops, buses, pubs, etc.; if you have to pass near someone keep 30 feet away; if you meet someone while out walking cover your nose with a handkerchief or step over a gate into a field until they have passed by. Not surprisingly the locals were initially mystified by such behaviour but soon came to understand why it was necessary.

The volunteers were told when they would be visited by staff and the arrangements for medical examinations; and how to find matron if they suddenly felt ill and the switchboard wasn't working—look for a flat with a red watering-can on the step. Food would be brought to them and they had to learn how to avoid making contact with those who were providing it. The importance of keeping the isolation rules was a constant theme. Anyone who, by accident or intent, turned up with a cold would already have been sent home. The first few days served as a quarantine period to uncover any who might be incubating a cold although showing no signs of this on arrival. Should a cold develop during this period the person concerned could stay on and complete the holiday or go home immediately and then make a return visit after the cold had gone.

Then they needed to know how to book a session of table tennis—only permissible with a flatmate—and how to sterilise the bat and ball when they were finished. They also heard what experiments were planned, such as tests for the effects of a new virus or a possible strain of vaccine or antiviral drug. They needed to know on which days they would have nose-drops, tablets, or sprays; and the general message was that these things would take up some time but were not dangerous or harmful. Proceedings were brought to a close with a short question-and-answer session. Then it was back to their flats to start working out how they were going to spend their days in this unusual holiday centre. They would not be enjoying any further lunches together or, indeed, any other communal activity, until the end of the trial.

Volunteers found various ways of coping with, or avoiding, the isolation rules. On one occasion two men discovered that a pair of young ladies occupied the adjacent flat in the other half of their hut. Quarantine restrictions had eliminated any internal link and a direct approach from outside would have

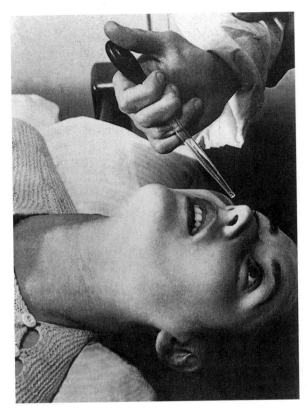

Fig. 7.4 Inoculation with nasal drops.

been observed. So how could they reach them without attracting attention? Any ex-prisoner of war would have found it laughably easy, and it did not take them long to find a solution. They noticed that the ceilings were made of loose roof panels—rather obvious since they bounced up and down as westerly gales swept across the downs. Moving some of these aside they climbed up into the roof space, crawled along, and descended into the next flat. However, this seems to have been a final act of defiance because they left the next day.

Dr Edward Lowbury, a unit bacteriologist in the early days, recalls quite a different problem posed by the isolation rules.

> One young man came with his girlfriend and, true to the conventions of the time, they were housed in separate flats. Like Romeo he would converse with her from a position below her balcony but always remaining beyond the minimum permitted distance of 30 feet. Then they asked if they could go for country walks provided they held a 30 ft piece of string taut between them. Permission was given and they

did their best to stay within the rules, but at an early stage things came unstuck, or rather they didn't. They attempted to pass either side of a tree, whereupon the string, still taut, folded back on itself, bringing its ends and the lovers together.

It was perfectly within the letter and spirit of the rules to have one's telephone plugged through to another flat and then to spend the evening playing chess with another like-minded volunteer. Conversations could be held by shouting between flats, either through adjacent windows or across whatever distance separated the huts, but such exchanges soon became tiring.

Most conformed with the rules but some tried outright disobedience. The local public houses were a huge temptation which a few were unable to resist. Unfortunately for them these were also frequented by members of staff. One bumped into the medical superintendent while heading for the nearby Rose and Crown. He was politely asked to come to the office next morning but had already packed his bags and gone by then. Another tried his luck in the next village, thinking that The Yew Tree in Odstock was sufficiently far away, only to find himself in the middle of a birthday celebration for two members of staff. But such breaches were most unusual—or extremely well-concealed. This was unsurprising in the circumstances. Everyone recognised that isolation was essential if the volunteer programme was to work. And the atmosphere was very relaxed. The medical officer, matron, and all the staff put the welfare of the volunteers first and spared no effort to make sure they were content. The small number who found the restrictions too much were simply given their marching orders, and their file cards suitably annotated.

Strict control of isolation was also helped by the irregular hours kept by members of staff. Some virology experiments lasted late into the night and anyone trying to slip quietly across to a neighbouring flat might well be confronted by a scientist strolling back from the laboratory. Whatever was alleged, there was never an organised programme of spying on volunteers, but resident staff were not discouraged from being vigilant.

Restricted rations

Wireless sets became part of the sitting room furniture from the outset, beginning with heavy valve sets that soon gave way to the more reliable and much lighter transistor receivers. Television followed as it became a normal part of life. I remember seeing black and white pictures of the coronation in New York in 1953. But sets were not available to the volunteers until the end of the decade, progressing over the years from pay-as-you-view to free, and from black and white to colour.

Social scientists believe that from the beginning of the twentieth century most people in Britain had four meals a day. Starting the day with breakfast, many men worked near their homes and could return for a meal at midday. Tea would follow at the end of the afternoon, and supper in the evening. Hospitals fed their patients on a similar pattern and we adopted the same regime at the CCU. Food rationing remained in force for some years after the war, placing severe restrictions on both quantity and choice. But these slowly relaxed and finally disappeared in 1954.

In the early years volunteers handed in their ration books so that the unit could buy the food and prepare it. The budget for this, set by the Ministry of Health, was initially based on what they reckoned to be adequate for feeding hospital patients. It was not enough. Our volunteers were mostly young and active and could not exist on a diet designed for an invalid. So an extra allowance was negotiated. Nevertheless the food had to be quite simple at first in order to keep within the ration and cost limits. A main meal included some sort of meat and vegetables, followed by a pudding; fruit and salads in season were provided; and there was bread and something to go on it—butter, margarine, or jam—enough, hopefully, to fill the stomachs of ravenous students. Later on there was much more variety. A full cooked breakfast would often come round in big thermos jugs, and there was cake at teatime followed by cold meats and perhaps cheese for supper.

The menus ran on a fairly predictable cycle but were not repeated during the course of a trial. And they were tailored to the wishes of volunteers where possible. A large blackboard on the kitchen wall carried messages such as 'Flat 3a vegetarian', or 'Flat 4b double potatoes' or 'Flat 6b no gravy'. It was a great tribute to the kitchen and to Tom, who did much of the purchasing, that many of the guinea pigs said how much they enjoyed the food, and some asked for the cook's recipes. In fact volunteers listed 'delicious meals' amongst memories of their visits. To a large extent the traditional diet was continued even when convenience foods became available and small ovens were installed in the flats. Ice cream had to be bought in but the chips were still home-made. The volunteers were not told the menu in advance so there was a certain sense of excitement as they came back from a morning walk or a game of ping-pong and picked up the thermos jug waiting at the door. What would it be today? The unit majored on such simple pleasures.

Honeymoons and suchlike

Two world wars had accelerated the emancipation of women. They had taken on jobs in factories and in the services that had previously been thought of as the preserve of men, and they drove ambulances and tractors. They also had to assume a wider responsibility for raising families than in peace time, though this was a normal role for wives of sailors and many soldiers. Statistics showed that the number of children born out of wedlock began to increase in the latter years of the war and the number of divorces rose too. This has led on to increasing numbers of one-parent families and step-children. But this had relatively little impact on the way the unit ran. For most men and women the basic expectation was that they would still only live together after they were married. Everyone knew that this was not universal but it was generally thought of as the 'right thing to do', and what the majority wanted and expected.

So the rules of the unit embodied these ideas. Single men or women were welcome. If they did not arrange to come with a friend to share the flat they were placed with someone who seemed likely to be compatible. In some cases this worked so well that the two who had been thrown together would repeat the arrangement the following year. Apart from family groups, a man and woman were only placed in the same flat if they were married to each other. And they might be only just married—that rarity we have already mentioned, the honeymoon couple. But there were no elaborate checks and no one asked for marriage certificates.

On some occasions romantic boy–girl emotions were stirred. It wasn't sur-prising—many of the young volunteers were good-looking, charming, and unattached. They were kept apart by the isolation rules until the end of the trial, but left the unit promising to keep in touch. Some did, at least for a while, but this rarely went on to finally tying the knot. Although public attitudes and practice had changed by the late 1980s, the rules remained and there was no demand for them to be altered. They were accepted as part of the picture. Perhaps the place was seen as a bit quaint and old-fashioned, but this was part of its charm, and in sharp contrast with the advanced nature of the science being practised there.

The range of volunteer amusements was limited only by the imagination and ingenuity of the individuals concerned, and the isolation rules. Almost everyone enjoyed walking along the lanes and footpaths of the surrounding countryside. This part of Wiltshire is a region of outstanding beauty, perfect for such a peaceful and relaxing form of exercise—except for one group which inadvertently blundered into the middle of a shoot on the nearby Longford Castle Estate and, as one of them put it, 'had to run like blazes'.

Practical jokes, inevitably, appealed to some of the more ruthless elements. Most were fairly harmless: misleading notes sent between flats, false announce-ments appearing on the notice board, and so on. Articles of clothing drying on a line frequently proved an irresistible target: underpants being sewn up, another pair being filled with jelly, and further variations on this theme. And it was not all one-way traffic. In the case of one local skirmish, retaliation was swift and effective. The victims of this particular prank discovered that their fuse box also served the adjacent flat where the perpetrators resided. The appropriate fuses were removed and the practical jokers spent their evening in darkness.

Knitting was popular amongst the ladies, the days of isolation contributing to some high production rates. Some made jam. Several had a job at writing poetry. One man serviced his car during the course of his stay. Another had timber delivered in order to build some units in his van. Evidently a persuasive sort of fellow, he also prevailed upon matron to make him some curtains.

A well-established routine

The largely unchanging pattern of social life amongst the volunteers was matched by the stability of the trial routine, which continued, with only minor adjustments, throughout the life of the unit. Many age groups were represented over the years but it was the young, and students in particular, who came in the largest numbers. One trial, which took place towards the end

Table 7.1

Day	Breakfast	Lunch	Supper
Monday		Lamb chops, potatoes,vegetables	
Tuesday	Cereal	Roast turkey, potatoes, vegetables	Cold meat salad
	Eggs	Fruit crumble & custard	Fresh fruit
Wednesday	Cereal	Steak & mushroom pie, potatoes, vegetables	Sausage & chipped potatoes
	Bacon & tomato	Ice cream & chocolate sauce	Jelly
Thursday	Cereal	Liver & bacon, potatoes, vegetables	Scotch fritters & baked beans
	Fish cakes	Fruit pie & custard	Cheese & biscuits
Friday	Cereal	cod au gratin, potatoes, vegetables	Welsh rarebit, bacon
	Sausage & tomato	Trifle	Fresh fruit
Saturday	Cereal	Cottage pie, potatoes, vegetables	Casseroles or salad
	Kippers	Fruit in jelly	Cheese & biscuits
Sunday	Cereal	Roast beef, Yorkshire pudding, potatoes, vegetables	Cold meat salad
	Bacon & eggs	Fruit crumble & cream	Fresh fruit
Monday	Cereal	Chicken chasseur, potatoes, vegetables	Pizza
	Bacon & beans	Bread & butter pudding	Blancmange
Tuesday	Cereal	Braised steak, potatoes, vegetables	Savoury mince, jacket potato
	Eggs	Bakewell tart	Cheese & biscuits
Wednesday	Cereal	Boiled gammon, potatoes, vegetables	Cold meat salad
	Sausage & tomato	Apple Charlotte & custard	Fresh fruit
Thursday	Cereal	Roast pork, apple sauce, potatoes, vegetables	Cold meat salad
	Bacon & fried bread	Gateau	Cheese & biscuits

of the 1980s, will serve as an example. There were 22 volunteers, 13 of them female, ranging in age from 18 to 49, but most were in their twenties and early thirties. Seven were students. The others represented a variety of occupations, including nursing, teaching, instrument technology, market research, computers, marine engineering, radiography, and panel-beating. And there was one young married couple who, I am quite certain, would not have been on honeymoon. These were much more affluent times.

Meals had become more varied since the days of rationing and, whilst sticking to fairly simple recipes, were sustaining and substantial, as the 'bill of fare' shown in the Table 7.1 suggests.

The trial procedure imposed some restrictions upon the volunteers' movements, since they had to be in their rooms at those times when tests were to be carried out, the frequency of the tests varying from day to day. But apart from these they were free to come and go as they wished, as long as they observed the no-contact rules. It was a fairly benign regime.

A little help from our friends

Help and advice was offered to us from all directions, and was certainly not confined to those intrepid people who came to serve as guinea pigs. Everyone has a view on colds and what to do about them, and we received a stream of letters offering us the most intriguing suggestions. Some of these came from journalists but most were from members of the general public. They arrived by the score, especially after some publicity. One of the duties of the medical superintendent was to deal with enquiries and suggestions about the unit, and he ensured that all of them were answered. Representative files of these survive from as far back as the 1940s and provide a fascinating insight into what people thought at that time.

Some wrote to get an expert second opinion on a health problem. This was often something to do with catarrh, sinusitis, or polyps, or possibly a nasal allergy. Other letters, from people who were clearly hypochondriacs, ran for many pages and included a great deal of circumstantial, but probably irrelevant, detail. We tried to help them and hoped that our replies would give them a nudge in the right direction, but often they were hoping for the sort of answers we could not provide. The unit had been set up to search for the cause of colds; we were not ready to look for or evaluate treatments.

This question of treatments was a continuing problem because that was what many of the letters were about. People offered to come to the unit so that we could investigate their case. But we wanted to study the viruses that we would give them rather than something they brought. Some correspondence

Table 7.2 Daily programme for trial of an antiviral spray

Tuesday	Clinical examination
	Blood – haematology, biochemistry, v.rapid neut.
	Nasal wash, C/R method – virus detection
	X-ray if necessary
	Enter isolation
	Psychology consent form & questionnaire
Wednesday	Urinalysis
	Clinical examination
	Nasal wash, C/R method & processing
	Performance test
	Practice sprays
	Psychology questionnaires 2 & 3
Thursday	Clinical examination
	Read v. rapid neut. 9 am & 5 pm
	Virus/saline challange 10 am & 11 am
Friday	Clinical examination
	Medication 8 am, 11 am, 2 pm, 5 pm, 8 pm, & 10.30 pm
Saturday	Clinical examination
& Sunday	Nasal wash, virus detection
	Medication 8 am, 11 am, 2 pm, 5 pm, 8 pm, & 10.30 pm
Monday	Clinical Examination
	Nasal wash, virus detection
	Performance test
	Medication 8 am, 11 am, 2 pm, 5 pm, 8 pm, & 10.30 pm
Tuesday	Clinical examination
	Nasal wash, Virus detection
	Medication 8 am, 11 am, 2 pm, 5 pm, 8 pm, & 10.30 pm
Wednesday	Clinical examination
	Nasal wash, virus detection
Thursday	Urinalysis
	Clinical examination
	Nasal wash, virus detection
	End isolation
	Blood – haematology & biochemistry

Convalescent sample of blood required from all volunteers
Volunteers to return 'cold report cards'

told us about methods that the writers or their families used to prevent or treat colds. Many of them reflected folk remedies or medical beliefs which had flourished in previous years and were still very much alive in some people's minds. One letter came from China, complete with tablets containing antler horn. Others told us that the best way to treat colds was with hot drinks, sweetened with honey or fruit juices, often laced with alcohol in various forms. Many seemed sensible and realistic, but we were looking for causes at this stage, not cures, and so all we could do was to keep such letters on file.

Quite a number of correspondents were confident that they knew how to prevent colds. Garlic was a favourite. The main idea was to swallow it in various forms, but rubbing it on one's socks was also considered benefi-cial—possibly by keeping cold sufferers out of sneezing range! Onions were also favoured, as well as various herbs. Some with more Spartan tendencies recommended regular cold baths as a toughening process.

Home-grown treatments were always popular—in some cases, one suspects, the more bizarre the better. I had a continuing correspondence with a gentleman who for 30 years has treated colds by inserting 2 or 3 mm of Cetavlon (a skin antiseptic that comes in a tube and is squeezed out like toothpaste) into the nostril as soon as it begins to run, repeating this for an hour and at bedtime. He claimed that this cures the cold 'in nearly all cases' but admitted that he had not persuaded his family to follow his example.

As I have already suggested, the greater the number of proposed remedies for a condition, the less likely it is that any of them are any good. But what is it that makes so many sane people think they are? Timing could well be the answer. Colds come and go frequently, varying in their intensity and, as we mentioned earlier, not always developing fully. Sometimes they produce a few mild symptoms and then disappear completely. If a particular treatment is used at such a time it is easy to think that this has prevented the onset when in fact the cold was going to abort anyway. People may go through periods in their lives when they have a lot of colds, followed by spells when they have hardly any. The likelihood is that the colds they suffered have provided them with a strong army of antibodies which are keeping them relatively immune to further attack—at least until something very different comes along. If their treatment coincides with this cold-free period then they will naturally see it as an effective remedy.

Individual attitudes can also be a factor. Some people are proactive in their response to life, preferring to make things happen rather than let things happen to them. Such people are less inclined to accept that a cold should attack them without anything being done about it. They want to take some action that will bring it to an end. They feel better for doing this, which is in accord with their nature, and they will naturally believe that their actions are having a positive effect.

Scientists are familiar with this situation when they first get an idea for a study or the first promising result emerges from an experiment. This might come after months, even years, of research. It could be the answer they have been waiting for. It is also a highly dangerous moment in which they could allow their desire for a successful outcome to cloud their judgement. That is why they then repeat the work in a double-blind, controlled study, which prevents their personal enthusiasm affecting the results.

There is a paradox here. It was their enthusiasm that drove them on in the first place and brought them to this point. But as they stand on the brink of success they must subdue that enthusiasm and ensure that they employ what is aptly termed a clinical or objective approach to their work as they seek to confirm their results. Only then can they convince both themselves and their fellow scientists that their idea is objectively true.

The ethics of experiments on humans

Debates concerning the rights and wrongs of research on human beings figured prominently during the life of the unit, and rightly so. Attitudes have changed since the nineteenth century and have led to a refinement in our approach in recent years. Nevertheless some of the basic principles were hammered out centuries ago. Physicians at the time of Hippocrates were expected to learn what they could about diagnosis and treatment, and this was what they claimed, or professed, as a member of a 'profession'. But the privileges they received as a learned profession were balanced by their responsibilities to act honourably and honestly towards each other and for the benefit of their patients. They were to be moral and altruistic. Such professional ethics have remained to the present day.

When volunteer experiments in cold research were started in the 1930s and again in 1946 the work was conducted by medically qualified people who believed it was their duty to ensure the health and welfare of the volunteers. Ultimate responsibility lay with the doctor in charge, and this responsibility was shared by the director of the MRC Institute, who knew about the experiments and had approved them.

Another issue was that of 'informed consent'. In 1830 Wilcock, in his book *Law relating to the medical profession*, wrote that provided the subject was told an experiment was proposed and he gave his consent, then the practitioner was not 'answerable...in damages'. In practice this means that the patient has not only to be informed of what is proposed but must also clearly understand its consequences. Medical practitioners ignored such rules at their peril.

Amauer Hansen, the famous Norwegian physician and worker on leprosy, was dismissed from his post because he inoculated leprosy bacilli into the eye of a patient without telling her what he was doing or getting her permission. Similarly, Hideyo Noguchi, of the Rockefeller Institute in New York, who was mentioned earlier, inoculated patients in a public hospital with an experimental skin test material without getting their permission, even though the material might have transmitted syphilis.

These things should not have happened because, by that time, the early twentieth century rules governing such situations had already been laid down. Formulated in Prussia, they stated that the subjects should give formal consent, their autonomy should be respected, and the experimenters should ensure that no harm was done. Yet this advice was not widely known or followed. In Germany and the English-speaking world drug trials were done without any of the ethical review and supervision that we expect today.

When the MRC proposed to inoculate volunteers with influenza virus in 1930, it was given a legal opinion that it would not be liable, provided consent was obtained. In the experiments on common colds, Andrewes was asked whether the experiments would give useful results and how much they would cost. The hospital said they must use pre-clinical students as otherwise students with colds might bring infection onto the wards. The students would go to a talk by Andrewes and could then apply to take part in the experiments. But there was no statement that the proposal was ethical (though it certainly was) or that it had been reviewed by any formal independent committee, as would be required today. Ethics were certainly recognised as important, but were not discussed in any formal way. It was simply understood that any project must take them into account.

The rules of war

War tends to produce its own rules or modifications of existing rules. And there must have been many experiments where there is no record of how individual consent was obtained. This is not to suggest there was anything unethical about the experiments, simply that regulations had not been firmly established, and those that had were not necessarily followed to the letter. Scientists tended to set their own ethical standards. For example, if they found a chemical that might be useful in treatment they would try it out on themselves and if it did them no harm they went ahead to use it on patients.

My own ideas concerning volunteers and medical research may have been influenced by some of my early experiences in Sheffield in the 1940s. In those days it was not unusual to be invited to take part in physiological experiments, and I remember how one of these made my heart pound violently while another gave me a severe pain in the arm. In the first instance, certainly, I do not think I was told what to expect.

It was also in Sheffield that I first saw experimentation with large numbers of volunteers. Close to the university where I was studying was a house full of these volunteers, recruited from the ranks of conscientious objectors by a certain Dr Kenneth Mellanby, son of Sir Edward Mellanby who was in charge at the MRC. A lecturer in zoology, Mellanby was looking for a way to control scabies, a skin disease which was causing a lot of trouble in air-raid shelters and in the armed forces. His volunteers, all men, were required to sleep in close proximity to each other in blankets contaminated with the causative mite. From this he was able to discover that there was no transmission from the blankets and that infestation was caused only by skin-to-skin contact. It was an important finding which, as Mellanby pointed out in a book he wrote after the war, could not have been discovered using animals. He found his volunteers to be so willing and cooperative that he recommended setting up a permanent station where they could take part in other important experiments conducted by visiting scientists.

At the end of the war the world learned of the ghastly experiments carried out by Nazi doctors in the concentration camps of wartime Germany. This resulted in a statement by judges at the Nuremberg trials, usually called the Nuremberg Code, which contains most of the rules to be observed when conducting experiments on humans. Since then it has been modified and refined in a series of further documents, the Helsinki Declaration being one of these.

The era of Nazi war crimes seems worlds away from the work of the CCU. But we were open to charges of bad practice. There were groups who held strong views, asserting that all experiments on humans were immoral and that clinical researchers were heartless people. And so there was a risk that volunteers would not come forward or that our work would be stopped. We had to be open about what we were doing and about what happened to volunteers. But there was no doubt about the importance of our work and most people recognised this. The CCU was set up for regular systematic research on a health problem of the nation. The ethical basis was that of good medical practice. This was clearly understood, and Andrewes and his director accepted responsibility for deciding what experiments were permissible.

We were clear that in recruiting volunteers, and experimenting on them and with them, we were engaging with fellow human beings in a joint enterprise, and we took care to ensure that the way in which we operated reinforced this feeling. It was sometimes thought that people who did research had to be inhuman and not care about individuals. Such views would colour people's reactions whenever there was a suspicion that the rules might not be observed. There were protests in the local papers when it became known in Harrow that, in 1970, the new district hospital was going to be linked with a research centre and that the staff would be looking after patients. In the event the only comments that came my way were on how humanely the patients were treated.

The rise of the 'Ethical Committee'

In 1963, Maurice Papworth, a physician well known for his excellent scheme of coaching young doctors for higher examinations in clinical medicine, wrote a book entitled *Human guinea pigs*. In this he gave a long and rather repetitive list of medical studies, mainly carried out on patients in academic departments of medicine. Many had already been published by medical journals. But he pointed out that seriously ill patients had been put through rigorous and invasive procedures as part of a research protocol, and not to assist in their diagnosis or treatment. There was little or no evidence that this had been explained to them or that anyone had asked their permission.

Papworth argued that the medical practitioners had been exploiting their position and the patients' trust. The procedures that he criticised, such as intravenous pyelography for X-rays of the kidneys, and cardiac catheterisation for the anatomy and functioning of the heart, are now used routinely because they are such valuable and informative investigations. But over a decade had passed since Nuremberg and medical research had done little to clarify or regulate its practices. The book was intended to rouse public indignation, and that it certainly did.

In the USA in the late 1950s a Dr Henry Beecher had also been campaigning on the same issues. Even by then a number of American institutions had still not adopted the Nuremberg Code and Beecher, who had worked on anaesthesia in human subjects, found a series of examples of unethical practice in the literature. His conclusions were opposed by colleagues who thought he was interfering and slowing up research, and it was probably they who made it difficult for him to get his papers published. One of his most contentious examples was the work of Saul Krugman, who had studied hepatitis virus infections in an institution for the care of mentally defective children.

After much drafting and redrafting there was enough agreement for the Declaration of Helsinki to be published by the World Medical Association in 1965. Meanwhile, the MRC had decided not to wait for this and in 1963 published its own guidelines covering experiments on human beings.

The CCU, of course, was expected to follow these rules, and it was not difficult to do so. Our experiments involved giving viruses that caused mild illness in humans, making simple observations, and collecting small samples of blood, nasal fluids, and urine. And we limited the freedom of movement of our volunteers by our isolation rules. All this was harmless. The point was that we recruited them without any direct pressure. And they had to contact us after hearing about the place, not the other way round. Their payment consisted of travel expenses and a very small amount of pocket money. Admittedly they were given their board and lodging, but all these things added together would hardly be a sufficient inducement to come against their better judgement. They were informed in writing about the experiments that were planned and had to send in a written application to attend. On arrival at the unit they were reminded of the nature of the experiments face to face and told they could leave at any moment. So by the time the studies actually started they had been well informed and their agreement to take part could be regarded as 'informed consent'.

CCU adopts ethical code

We determined that we must have a formal ethical review of the experiments we were planning, and it happened that certain organisational changes made this a more straightforward matter. Previously we had been part of the NIMR but the MRC was setting up a Clinical Research Centre at Harrow in 1967 and this became our supervisory body. The NHS authorities had also established an independent ethical committee at Harrow to review research being done in the Northwick Park Hospital. And so whenever we were planning new types of experiments or studies using novel materials we first sent our proposals to this committee for review.

Its first step was to get an opinion from a scientific advisory committee on two important criteria: did the research address a significant scientific question and was it designed to produce results that were capable of giving a valid answer. This scientific group could be helpful in picking out some flaw in the design, perhaps in the statistics, and this could be rectified before the application went forward. It was an excellent discipline that ensured each new research project was justified, down to the finest detail. As was pointed out, 'even the taking of a blood sample without good reason is not ethical'.

The process was not as cumbersome as it may sound. The main points of the experiment were readily transferred to the application form, and this was dealt with quickly so research was not held up. If anyone later expressed doubts about the work it was reassuring to know that the protocols had been reviewed independently and considered to be ethical. We also helped the committee to monitor what was going on by sending it reprints of papers published as a result of work that it had reviewed.

We were happy with the way things worked. Apparent conflicts could be avoided or resolved provided there were clear guidelines and everyone was kept informed. But such problems are certain to increase rather than diminish as further advances are made, particularly in the field of molecular genetics. It would need the input of various people—clinicians, scientists, counsellors and ethicists—to make the issues clear to everyone concerned and then resolve them in a way that takes into account all the major principles of the contributors to the debate. This would take time and might require additional research but it is well worth the effort. We must retain the optimal way to treat our fellow human beings as learned over past centuries and apply it conscientiously as we confront the new knowledge about our genes. And in so doing we may benefit our fellows in ways that could barely be imagined a few decades ago.

CHAPTER 8

International cooperation

Diseases travel the world, taking no note of boundaries. They are the true internationals, and we have to deal with them accordingly. Some have a preference for a particular region, perhaps thriving in warmer climes, but the majority have no such limitations. And of these the common cold must surely be the most ubiquitous international of them all. We needed to pursue this experienced traveller as far as we could by having an international dimension to our own studies. For example, were the rhinoviruses found in Salisbury causing colds abroad?

The new cold viruses that we had discovered needed to be studied in detail. There were also other viruses that had been found in lower respiratory diseases of infants, such as pneumonia and certain forms of bronchiolitis. Some of these, such as parainfluenza viruses, could infect volunteers and produce illnesses that were clinically just like colds seen in the community. We also needed to know which viruses caused the outbreaks of colds we have every winter. Do similar viruses occur around the world or do they vary from place to place? Are there waves of new viruses sweeping across the globe, as happens periodically with influenza?

Christopher Andrewes had played a key role in the early days of WHO and so, in 1946, the World Influenza Centre was sited in his department. He saw it as an effective way to make contact with others working on the same problems and to organise collaborative studies when needed. WHO continues to do this, and the eradication of smallpox in 1977 and expert meetings on AIDS and BSE are more recent examples of this international approach.

In 1960 Andrewes decided that it would be a good idea to constitute the CCU as a WHO reference laboratory for respiratory viruses on the model of the influenza laboratories. This would provide the international contacts that would enable us to identify the different serotypes and investigate the epidemic spread of these new viruses. His first step was to persuade the MRC to recognise the unit as a respiratory virus group and to pay for an increased staff. He then wrote with his usual enthusiasm to his contact at WHO in Geneva, putting the idea to him. But once again his eagerness to get things done had led him into a tactical error: he failed to go through the correct MRC channels and was duly reprimanded by his seniors.

It was only a temporary setback. The idea was recognised as a potentially valuable one and in due course his proposal was supported. A formal agreement was drawn up giving the unit status as a WHO laboratory with a small amount of financial support. It was the start of a long collaboration.

WHO had a clearly defined role with regard to reference laboratories and described this in its introduction to a report on the first years of the influenza programme.

> Fundamental research and the development of new techniques, at least in their initial stages, are best carried out through private or institutional initiative. The role of WHO is to facilitate this work by various means: collecting and distributing epidemiological and laboratory findings on an international scale; promoting the rapid exchange of scientific information among the various workers throughout the world; providing for training of specialised workers; and providing standard diagnostic reagents and other laboratory needs.

A confusion of names and numbers

WHO recognised the importance of collecting information on health matters from all corners of the globe and then ensuring that this reached people with the knowledge and skills to do something about it. Initially this might be no more than comparing reports, noting trends, and recording information. But eventually it led to the forecasting of epidemics, the development of treatments and, in some cases, to the eradication or control of a disease, either worldwide or in specific regions.

The purpose of the new group was to speed up the understanding of acute respiratory diseases and to use this knowledge to improve human health. Other laboratories besides Salisbury were also designated, and regular meetings between their directors were begun. As one of the directors involved, I found that this part went particularly smoothly as it meant conferring with a number of people I already knew quite well.

The WHO respiratory virus laboratory for the United States was at the National Institutes of Health (NIH), Bethesda, Maryland, under Dr R. M. (Bob) Chanock, and he and I had worked together in the past. Chanock came from Chicago, Illinois, where his mother was a concert pianist and his father a successful businessman. Graduating in medicine there and training in paediatrics, he then studied infections under Albert Sabin in Cincinnati, Ohio. After this apprenticeship he moved to the National Institute of Allergy and Infectious Diseases on the NIH site at Bethesda, where he remained for the rest of his professional career. A dynamic individual, Chanock built up a large and productive research group. Amongst the projects he initiated was a successful programme to look for viruses in children, admitted to hospitals in the Washington area, who were suffering from a variety of respiratory infections. But his team also looked for live influenza virus vaccine strains and studied viruses of diarrhoea.

We had cooperated in the study of parainfluenza viruses isolated in Europe and shown that they caused colds and similar illnesses in volunteers. In parallel with this we also studied the exact relationship of our viruses to the original strains isolated at the NIH. Viruses, blood samples, and information were exchanged and we compared results. It was a straightforward exercise, and we obtained fairly clear-cut answers. But in the case of these new common cold viruses the difficulties were much greater.

We sent our strains to the NIH and gave advice on how to grow them in the laboratory. Very quickly they were isolating their own strains and it became clear that there were two major problems. One was that these viruses were very much like poliovirus and the related enteroviruses. But were they similar enough to be categorised with them? We did not think so and felt that they should be identified as a new and separate group under the heading of rhinoviruses. The differences seemed crucial, particularly in the conditions required to grow them and the fact that they were readily inactivated by weak acids, whereas enteroviruses were acid resistant. However, some enterovirus experts considered that the similarities were so important that they should be added to the enterovirus family and given enterovirus numbers.

Andrewes and others argued the case for a separate group at scientific meetings. Now only a few years from retirement Andrewes was still an important figure in the growing field of virus taxonomy, and his views carried considerable weight. Chanock and I supported the thesis with a very careful description of what we saw as typical rhinoviruses. This was not rushed into print but sent to various virologists and reviewed by a 'parliament' of enterovirologists, the Picornavirus Taxonomy Committee under J. L. (Joe) Melnick, Director of a WHO reference laboratory on enteroviruses. The concept was presented most diplomatically to those who disagreed and, eventually, it was accepted that the separation made sense. So there was now a group of pico (little) viruses containing RNA—picornaviruses. And this had two subgroups: enteroviruses that lived in the intestine and rhinoviruses that lived in the nose.

The second problem was of a different kind and would take a good deal more time to sort out. Although we could now do a few tests and show that we had a rhinovirus in a specimen, we had found this to be only part of the story. Different human and animal sera neutralised some viruses but not others. The viruses had different antigens on their surfaces. These serotypes would have to be sorted out if we were to understand them properly, and that would be a huge task. We had to work out how many serotypes of rhinoviruses there were and give them all agreed numbers.

Viruses were being grown from patients in a number of areas: in Britain, at the CCU, in Public Health Laboratory Service, and university labs; and in the USA, at centres such as NIH, the University of Chicago, and in the laboratories of Merck Sharp and Dohme (where they were called coryzaviruses). All were designated by numbers and letters in a very confusing way, and it was not clear whether there were many different viruses or a few viruses with many different names.

Studying the epidemiology and spread of the organisms was impossible under these conditions. We could not even make a start. WHO were brought into the picture once more and agreement was reached on using its network for a collaborative serotyping programme, following the pattern of the one already started on enteroviruses. Various labs would be asked to provide a small number of apparently 'new' strains, representative of what they had found. Each would be 'purified' by passing at limiting dilution, and a pool of this virus would be used to prepare an anti-serum in a laboratory animal. All the viruses would then be tested against all the sera. The work would be spread between the collaborating labs, but in the NIH all the tests would be repeated in a single laboratory.

Bring on the goats

At Salisbury the main task was given to a recently recruited scientist, Dr Paul Chapple, mentioned earlier, and his technician. This took up a substantial proportion of our resources but other laboratories contributed more, particularly in the USA. We were at some disadvantage in relation to our American friends: they could buy-in commercially prepared tissue cultures but we had to make all our own. We also had to develop, from scratch, methods of producing large volumes of culture fluids and then 'clean up' the virus they contained. Making enough serum for the whole collaboration, against the viruses allocated to us, was another substantial task.

We could not use human serum because this would already contain antibodies resulting from earlier virus attacks. The animal kingdom, however, is not susceptible to the viruses that interested us and so would be free of the relevant antibodies. Injection of such a virus into an animal would cause it no discomfort—it would not be aware that anything had happened—but its immune system would still produce the appropriate antibodies. So the serum from this animal would provide a means of identifying the virus on future occasions. It was just a question of which animal to use. We decided on goats.

A strange choice, perhaps, but goats have their advantages. They are hardy creatures, need very little care, will eat almost anything, and would certainly enable us to produce the required volume of serum. We had plenty of space but needed to build pens for them. Unfortunately our decision to do this coincided with exceptional winter conditions. These were the early weeks of 1963 and the country was locked in an unprecedented depth of snow and ice. The acquisition of goats had to be put on hold for a few weeks, but the delay was something we found difficult to explain to colleagues in the mid-western states of America where they regularly had months of snow in the winter, without it bringing the chaos we experienced.

Eventually the weather relented; we built our pens, and bought our goats. They were pleasant, if slightly wilful, animals who soon became part of the family—almost literally as it turned out. The reason was that the members of our staff responsible for looking after them did not usually come in at week-ends, but the animals still had to be fed. And so my family took on the task—not unwillingly, I should add, the children loved the idea. The arrangement worked well except when one of the goats felt obliged to live up to its reputation and consumed a sizeable portion of one child's sweater.

Serum production was soon meeting demand once we had brought the goats on stream. We also assisted other laboratories by 'purifying' some coryzaviruses and freeze-dried numerous strains to help in their conservation and distribution. Tedious and exacting work, but in the end hundreds of results were available and could be collated.

Al Kapikian, who ran the central tests at NIH, visited Salisbury in July 1966 to discuss the results of the WHO collaboration with Andrewes and CCU staff. And at this point the numbering system for the first 55 serotypes was proposed. Kapikian then went on to Moscow to present the outcome at a meeting of directors of WHO laboratories, where the group's findings were endorsed and passed on to the International Committee for Virus Nomenclature.

I was impressed to find that the labs gave their help in a most unselfish way and that the results of the duplicate tests were in close agreement. Much of the expense fell upon the American laboratories.

Numerous viruses had still to be tested and classified, and these formed the subject of two further programmes, this time under the chairmanship of

Vince Hamparian (previously of Merck Sharp and Dohme). These succeeded in defining a total of 100 serotypes. There may well be more but at the moment there is little enthusiasm for further work of this sort. Part of the reason lies in differing concepts of the role and epidemiology of the rhinoviruses that have been emerging.

Collaboration with the WHO network went extremely well whenever there was a need for this kind of cooperation. But much of our work was pursued independently, as was that of other WHO reference laboratories. For example, NIH used their own network for defining the nature of *Mycoplasma pneumoniae*, the cause of primary atypical pneumonia and previously thought of as a respiratory virus. Similarly, we continued to define and name newly recognised viruses; and we did much of the work in recognising some human coronaviruses as a further cause of colds, at the same time establishing their relationship to viruses of birds and mice. However, in this context, we were very grateful to Dorothy Hamre at the University of Chicago for sending us her virus and for Al Kapikian's help in confirming our results and getting agreement to our ideas from bird and mouse virologists in the USA.

WHO ideas expand

WHO quickly realised that this network of virus disease reference laboratories could adopt a wider role than that initially set for them. In 1961 a WHO scientific group on virus diseases proposed that the laboratories should also anticipate and define problems of international public health and advise on laboratory and field problems. After a further triennial review it was stated in 1967 that they were also to encourage laboratory and field research 'necessary for the prevention and control of disease'. In 1974, after a similar review, there was more emphasis on WHO taking the initiative. In future the laboratories were to be known as WHO Collaborative Centres for Reference and Research, and they were charged with taking an active part in collaborative field and laboratory studies set up by WHO. The number of centres increased substantially, many of them with special expertise in a much wider range of scientific subjects.

Thus the scope and emphasis of the CCU and the other centres changed gradually over the years. Although largely in response to the increase in scientific knowledge, these also reflected changes in the official views in Geneva concerning the type of work in which WHO should engage. In 1960 there was an opportunity to apply the new techniques in some important areas: in the search for new cold viruses; to establish how many different viruses there are; and to identify the diseases in which they are to be found. This meant focusing on bench procedures and reagents. It took time, and in some meetings members protested that we were simply concentrating on ivory tower science and doing nothing to improve the world's health. I particularly remember Herdis von Magnus from Copenhagen expressing this view at a meeting in London. She was experienced in public health virology and was probably more sensitive to the needs of developing countries than were a number of the group at the time.

But a start had been made in applying laboratory methods to health problems overseas. A 1967 serological study of children admitted to hospital with lower respiratory disease in countries around the world indicated that infection with viruses, like respiratory syncytial virus and parainfluenza viruses, first found in Washington, DC, were also important elsewhere. Studies in Salisbury showed that antibodies against viruses common in Britain—parainfluenza viruses, rhinoviruses and so on—were also common in sera collected in many parts of the world. It might well be that cold viruses were really common everywhere. On the whole they did not seem to be dangerous in developed countries. But to what extent were the newly discovered viruses responsible for the millions of deaths from respiratory infections that were occurring among children in developing countries each year? This was a question we certainly needed to answer.

Health for all by the year...?

'Health for all by the year 2000' was a slogan widely adopted following a momentous meeting on primary healthcare which took place in Alma Ata, southern Kazakhstan, in 1978. The mood was changing, and there was a feeling that something dramatic had to be done. Already in 1976 the World Health Assembly had instructed WHO to consider measures for combating the millions of deaths caused by acute respiratory infections in children under five. WHO responded with a one-week meeting of the Scientific Group on Virus Diseases in Geneva in September 1977. Staff from the Tuberculosis and Respiratory Unit of WHO were then brought in to work with members of the centres in order to speed the process of setting up the early studies.

It was clear that for a proper estimate of the clinical pattern and causes of such illnesses it would be necessary to study groups of sick children in poor environments such as rural villages and urban slums. This was where the clinical problems were to be found. The patients would be classified clinically and samples collected to be tested for possible virus and bacterial infections. The specimens needed were secretions aspirated from the nose and throat, a method which had been well-developed and was well-tolerated by the patients.

Immunofluorescence techniques would be employed to look for cells infected with viruses such as respiratory syncytial virus, parainfluenza, and influenza. Such tests could be set up in laboratories in many developing countries, and their sensitivity and specificity could be checked by sending some duplicates to various WHO reference laboratories. Where possible some of the specimens would also be tested for virus isolation. Although it was difficult to find satisfactory methods of testing for pathogenic bacteria, such organisms were also cultured.

At the same time a careful search was made for all the scattered papers on acute respiratory infections in children under five in developing countries. Surprisingly, although the results were not always strictly comparable, the figures indicated that the overall frequency of illnesses of all grades was similar to that in industrialised countries. Yet there were far more cases of fatal lower respiratory diseases, such as pneumonia, in children in developing countries. Virus infection did not seem to be the whole answer. There had to be other factors.

There were relatively few studies using strict criteria, such as recovery of organisms by blood culture or lung puncture, but these showed that bacteria such as pneumococci and *Haemophilus influenzae* were of major importance. Indeed the group working in Papua New Guinea had shown that the cases they saw were often due to pneumococci and responded well to penicillin. The literature showed that lack of breast feeding, malnutrition, and smoke pollution were probable risk factors. There was also evidence that in developing countries children had very high carrier rates of pneumococci and other bacteria, and this might also increase the chance of bacterial pneumonia occurring so frequently and so early in life. Pneumococci are generally found in the upper respiratory tract and are responsible for pneumonia, sinusitis, and meningitis.

All this suggested that viruses were the cause of much illness but that bacterial infections were the killers.

A global attack on respiratory diseases

It was to be a worldwide survey, involving as many overseas territories as possible. A number of WHO reference centres had already investigated the role of viruses in common respiratory disease in their local communities, and so these new studies served as a follow-up to those earlier surveys. More importantly they provided an effective blueprint for the new project. We had done a study based on Public Health Laboratory Service virus laboratories in the UK at the beginning of the 1960s, and so, with staff from other centres, took part in preparing protocols for the overseas studies.

The WHO regional offices knew where to find groups of interested people in the selected regions who shared their objectives and were willing to be involved in setting up and running studies. I was a member of teams who met in Rio de Janeiro, Nairobi, and Beijing between 1979 and 1981 to plan studies in the local communities.

Gradually the details began to emerge and were published by WHO. The first to appear was *Viral respiratory diseases*, which outlined the current state of knowledge on the subject; and this was followed, in 1982, by *Guidelines for research on acute respiratory infections II*. Many of the studies recorded, for the first time, the size and nature of the problem in various communities around the world. But establishing the extent of the problem was just the first step. The most important part was still to come: the institution of a medical programme that would help to turn back the tide of disease that was threatening some of these countries. Indeed the urgency was by now so great that it was decided to introduce some measures even before the survey had been fully completed. In 1981 the first proposals for a healthcare scheme, based largely on what had already been discovered in places like Goroka in Papua New Guinea, were set out in *Clinical management of acute respiratory infections in children*.

The studies were difficult and laborious, taking longer in some regions than in others, but eventually all the results were analysed and made ready for scrutiny by the Technical Advisory Group. This group, which had been appointed to review the programme, met in 1983. The conclusions it reached were that the milder illnesses often yielded viruses; that the viruses found were similar to those detected in industrialised countries; that the most serious lower respiratory tract disease was due to bacteria such as pneumococci; and that those who suffered from such bacterial attack were often predisposed to it by conditions such as malnutrition or other chest or heart diseases. We now had solid evidence as to the nature of the problem, but in order to combat it we needed to devise a way of recognising those cases likely to be due to bacteria, and appropriate treatment had then to be developed.

First we had to know if case-finding, management, and treatment could be taught and implemented. Trials would have to be set up in realistic field conditions as before, but there would be little need for virological expertise; instead we would require paediatricians with experience in recognising severe respiratory illnesses in primitive situations and capable of teaching mothers, nurses, and village health workers how to do the same. The local bacterial strains would have to be studied to determine which antibacterial drug should be used. Then a protocol could be tried out, in which a community tackled the range of childhood colds and coughs by separating out those that could be given reassurance or simple symptomatic treatment; those to be given antibacterial drugs, such as cotrimoxazole; and the most severe cases that would be sent as fast as possible to a local clinic where oxygen, nursing, and other antibacterial measures could be deployed.

It was a huge task, fraught with difficulties. The right staff had to be recruited and trained, good records maintained, and the outcome monitored. One of the hardest aspects was to find a comparison or control group against which to measure objectively those improvements in health that were seen to be due to the effects of the programme. And WHO needed evidence that the simplified diagnosis could be learned and practised, and that the management would deliver effective treatment to those who needed it.

Eventually these components were put into place, although more effectively in some areas than in others. It was a long process, involving many people across the globe. But it was worth it for it showed clearly how the mortality from acute respiratory infections in children under five could be significantly reduced.

CCU plays a supporting role

Once the programme was up and running we played a supporting role during the period of clinical investigation. Frequently our help was in quite small, albeit essential, matters. In 1980 a study was taking place at Dong-Guan, a village in the People's Republic of China not far from Beijing. The material from the children was to be tested for viruses in the laboratories of the Capital Institute of Paediatrics and they wanted samples of the record cards we used in this country. The request was easily satisfied since my wife had some she used in her own work in community paediatrics. Specific reagents were also sent to them from Salisbury, with WHO arranging their transport through what was then described as the Bamboo Curtain.

A couple of years later we entertained one of their key researchers, a Dr Zhu Zhonghan, who had a shopping list of things he wished to study in England. Newcastle upon Tyne was his first port of call, where he spent time with Professor Dick Madeley to learn certain diagnostic methods—particularly those based on immunofluorescence—and to improve his spoken English. This was followed by a period in Salisbury to hear about some of the more recently discovered viruses. Dr Zhu was one of many scientists who came to learn about our work. I welcomed these visits as a means of spreading the knowledge we had acquired as widely as possible and thereby helping other countries in their work on respiratory diseases.

Particularly important was our involvement in Technical Advisory Group meetings, including the key meeting in 1983 which covered the reports of the acute respiratory infections programmes, research on symptomatic diagnosis, treatment, etc., and the current situation on the development of respiratory virus vaccines. The conclusions of this meeting on how WHO should proceed were embodied in a memorandum which was endorsed by the Advisory Committee on Medical Research and published in 1984. Also in 1984 there was an important international meeting, organised by the University of Adelaide, South Australia, at which much of the information was reviewed. It concluded with a strongly worded recommendation that WHO and other bodies should do something to get the acute respiratory infections healthcare scheme implemented in developing countries throughout the world.

Reducing infant mortality

Response to this WHO recommendation varied considerably but, by 1992, the acute respiratory infections programme was active on a wide scale. The Technical Advisory Group review reported that 88 countries were being targeted. Of these, local guidelines had been developed in 62, with national plans to implement them, and the scheme was operational in 47, though to a varying extent. But there were also 20 non-target countries which had plans working. Gradually there was evidence in some areas that introduction of the guidelines had lowered the death rate from severe acute respiratory infections.

The cost of all this was substantial, and WHO was having difficulty in meeting it. It had $2.1 million available from its own budget, supplemented by $5.8 million from other sources, mainly international bodies and industrialised nations. But even when adding in unspent funds from the previous year there were only $10.5 million available to meet obligations of $13.4 million for the coming year. Both the Technical Advisory Group and a Meeting of Interested Parties advised a review of how the money was being spent and were in favour of integrating the acute respiratory infections activities with those of the well-established programme called Control of Diarrhoeal Diseases.

This programme had begun at a time when attacks of diarrhoea killed more infants and young children than any other disease. Analysis of the problem threw up a surprisingly simple form of treatment—not a complete remedy but of considerable value and readily applied. It had been found that drinking mixtures of water and salts, already being used to save the lives of patients with cholera, would also benefit people suffering from diarrhoea. So the programme set out to introduce this to millions of homes, while continuing research on the subject. It showed mothers how to make up and use these simple solutions and the health statistics began to improve.

Integration seemed a sensible use of resources and so it was agreed to convert the two programmes into one called the Integrated Management of Childhood Illness. This is now being actively promoted and evaluated throughout the world. It is not a settled and static scheme: knowledge and health problems are always in flux, and those involved have to deal with a number of quite different needs. Methods employed in one type of illness are only rarely applicable in another. Laboratory and clinical monitoring will have to continue and some guidelines will no doubt be changed as a result. And research will still be needed to produce novel vaccines, particularly against the viruses involved in both respiratory infections and diarrhoea, such as respiratory syncytial virus, parainfluenza, and rotaviruses.

The aim is to train and resource health workers to manage both groups of diseases, but it needs to be shown that there are practical ways of doing this. Can the staff be trained in this way, the resources provided, and the care delivered effectively? And can it be done in a wide range of environments and at a sustainable cost? The work will take many years, assuming these questions can be answered, but if it succeeds it will improve care and save the lives of millions.

Meetings at the centre

Directors of the WHO virus reference centres normally met at least once a year in Geneva. Our first meeting took place in 1961 at the Palais des Nations, a stately building where proceedings were accompanied by the call of peacocks strutting the lawns outside. In later years we met in the new, purpose-built WHO headquarters building, where we occupied spacious high-tech chambers complete with booths for interpreters (who were never used by us). I remember that it also offered a splendid view of the Jura Mountains through the glazing that took up most of one wall.

All our meetings followed a similar pattern: a brief welcome by a representative of the director of WHO, the appointment of a chairman and vice-chairman, and the choosing of rapporteurs, who would record all the proceedings. Accompanying the invitation to each director had been a request to produce one or more working papers. And so the meetings began with each centre presenting a report on its work, with background papers covering both their own research and that of others in their field. Inevitably there would be a lot of statistics but these were essential if we were fully to update the meeting on a particular science around the world. In my case this might be the state of development of antiviral drugs or a study of newly discovered organisms, such as coronaviruses. There would also be reports on the work done in training scientists as visiting workers from other countries. The language throughout was English, making it particularly hard work for some of the members, though they never complained.

These meetings were different from most other scientific gatherings that I attended, being tightly structured and fully documented. Only small numbers were involved, and they cut through the barriers of politics and economics. WHO staff also prepared thorough working papers, and there would be the annual report of activities at the Geneva centre. Many of the meeting reports re-emerged as papers in the WHO Bulletin, or formed part of the technical report series, or appeared as WHO monographs, ensuring that the views of WHO experts were passed on to medical and public health workers around the world. It was also quite usual for other important scientific issues, not directly concerned with the work of those attending, to be discussed; and reports on these special subjects would be issued in the same way.

Virus research was the area in which we were all involved and it was being pushed along very fast, often by the very people attending the meeting. Each group would talk about the research in which it was engaged, the development of new techniques, and provide information on the nature, pathogenicity, or epidemiology of viruses in its area. Sometimes this was relevant to agreed WHO objectives, but at other times it enabled us to present work that was new and exciting and likely to interest both WHO and virologists in general. For instance, we were able to tell our colleagues about our studies into the effects of interferon and other antiviral drugs when these were not generally known.

WHO officials also contributed. They had analysed reports of infections around the world and found no evidence that the newly discovered viruses spread like influenza. Similar viruses seemed to be active everywhere, and the differences between different laboratory reports seemed to depend mainly on the types of cases they studied and how effectively or enthusiastically they searched for different viruses.

WHO, as an agency of the United Nations, has a global responsibility. It has to respond to the ever-changing pattern of disease and the advances of medical science in each continent; identify and harness the expertise and resources of different countries; and, particularly in those early days, had to tread a careful path through the political differences and antagonisms that divided the world. Many of these differences still remain, of course, but are not perhaps as serious as they were in the days of the Cold War and apartheid. When we met, good manners demanded that everyone was treated courteously, and political differences were not allowed to intrude too much. Occasionally these might show up in the form of excessive paperwork or a lack of cooperation between sections, but in general WHO stuck to its objectives, ignored the politics, and did an excellent job in what were sometimes difficult situations. Particularly important was its ability to push forward key research projects which might otherwise have progressed too slowly.

A matter of breeding

One such project concerned the possibility of developing a live influenza virus vaccine. And it illustrates how WHO could set aside formal structures when it needed to. We knew that a fresh pandemic could occur at any time. We also knew that a live vaccine might be more effective in combating it than the standard injected vaccine, containing killed virus. The problem was that previous attempts at producing a live vaccine had ended up with something more likely to cause the disease than provide immunity. Some people doubted that a suitable strain could be identified or produced. But, in the late 1950s, we had shown that a Russian strain, IKSHA, had the necessary properties. We then studied other candidate strains in our volunteers at the CCU and reported on this during informal discussions with WHO.

What we were trying to do was to combine elements of an epidemic virus with those of a more benign laboratory-produced virus which would then induce the desired immunity. Working with NIMR, we studied attenuated strains produced by cross-breeding the new epidemic viruses with laboratory strains, such as PR8 or OKUDA. These had been well adapted to eggs and were also harmless to man. Given as nose-drops they stimulated immunity against influenza.

At first it was not clear what happened when a 'wild' virus became a 'mild' virus. But then laboratory workers unravelled the structure of influenza viruses and their eight genes. And they could work out which genes weakened, or attenuated, the virus. Eventually they could produce a virus in which, say, the genes for the inside of the virus came from PR8, so it was attenuated, while the genes for the outside came from the current epidemic virus and would stimulate immunity.

The American approach was different. Rather than look for attenuated genes as the British workers had done, they used their skills in the manipulation of virus genes to make such viruses temperature sensitive so that they would only grow poorly at body temperature—well enough to produce immunity but not enough to cause disease. Unfortunately they proved to be unstable when given as a vaccine: once inside the body the temperature-sensitive characteristic was not maintained and the virus became virulent and capable of bringing on the disease it was intended to prevent.

Then, in the 1960s, both the Americans and the Soviets found 'master strain' viruses that had been grown repeatedly at low temperatures and now contained attenuated genes that did not become virulent when they grew in the body. They produced candidate vaccines by cross-breeding with epidemic viruses. The Americans had tried their vaccines out on a few volunteers, the Soviets on millions, apparently. Both said they conferred immunity but had used different methods of testing. Which was better, or were they equally good?

The obvious thing to do was to compare the vaccines side by side—but how? The Cold War was in progress and the Iron Curtain was a very real barrier. However, WHO arranged a meeting to review the science in detail and invited both the Soviets and the Americans to send samples of their vaccines to Geneva for comparison. This they agreed to do. Small stocks of each vaccine were then made in the UK by Wellcome Research Laboratories and safety-tested before being given to groups of volunteers at Salisbury and later to students at Leicester. Laboratory tests showed that the two vaccines were similar and would immunise without causing disease. But no product has yet been licensed.

The story is still running. Work continues in the laboratories and clinics of the United States. New ways of changing the virus genome have been used to produce attenuated vaccine strains quickly and confidently. Much of this confidence stems from early work at the CCU by Dr Paul Beare who showed independently that attenuated virus strains could be found and, with NIMR colleagues, demonstrated that this attenuation is linked with the virus genes. It is important that this work reaches a successful conclusion because we can produce much greater quantities of live vaccine than the standard inactivated vaccine. And in the event of a major epidemic or pandemic of influenza we would be able to protect many more people.

Beare had trained in medicine in Cork, Ireland and then began general practice in England. But the Second World War intervened and he was called up into the army, eventually becoming a consultant pathologist. His particular interest was infections and he furthered his knowledge of the subject by taking courses in virology at the army laboratories in Millbank, London. After the war he left the army and joined the pharmaceutical research and products company, Pfizer, in Kent where he worked for a while before joining the CCU. He was to provide us with valuable insights into the disciplines of certain types of drug trials.

New technology may well bring live influenza vaccine into clinical use within a few years, and I like to think that one useful ingredient in the early stages of the development was the networking and helpful collaboration between the WHO centres and the steady trial work of the CCU.

The human factors

The fact that WHO was able to surmount the formidable barriers of the Iron and Bamboo Curtains indicates the esteem in which it was held throughout the world. The contacts made under its auspices were of enormous value and usually quite easy to bring about. The head of the Virus Unit in Geneva often played a key role. For many years the man in question was W. C. (Charles) Cockburn, a mild-mannered and friendly Scot who had trained as an epidemiologist and came to WHO from a post in the Public Health Laboratory Service.

Cockburn ran a smooth and disciplined organisation but could also be an opportunist when the situation demanded it. At a meeting in Leiden, before the WHO reference laboratories were designated, Bob Chanock mentioned over dinner that he wished to find out if the different CCU and NIH methods for measuring rhinovirus antibodies gave comparable results. He wanted David Taylor-Robinson, the first person to show there are different serotypes of rhinoviruses, to come to the NIH and do the crucial experiments. No problem: Cockburn arranged the move, with little or no formality, as soon as he returned to Geneva.

This unofficial arrangement had an interesting sequel and provides further evidence of how chance plays its part in our lives. Taylor-Robinson successfully completed the experiments for which he went to NIH and then took part in early work cultivating *Mycoplasma pneumoniae*. This is a cell-associated bacterium, thought at the time to be a virus. He never looked back: he did very little more work on viruses and became a world authority on mycoplasmas. I am sure Cockburn was pleased that he inadvertently launched him in this way.

Early in the 1980s, Cockburn was followed as head of the Virus Unit by a man of quite different character. Fakhry Assaad, an Egyptian, had trained partly in the UK and then worked for WHO on the epidemiology of trachoma in Taiwan, incidentally adding Mandarin Chinese to the various other languages in which he was fluent. This remarkable man, broadly built with a shock of grey hair, was a shrewd judge of people, with an outgoing personality and the ability to make everyone feel welcome and valued at meetings. He had a deep understanding of infectious diseases. I remember him saying, when AIDS had just been recognised and was thought to be a local problem mainly for North America, that it would have worldwide implications in which WHO should get involved. Tragically, at the height of his considerable powers, Fakhry Assaad was struck down with pneumonia which turned out to be secondary to an untreatable leukaemia. His death was a huge loss to us all.

Reflections

Documents, letters, and publications from the past show that much of what happened at the CCU was not foreseen, though some of the original ideas did work out as anticipated. It was eventually possible to hunt down cold viruses by using human volunteers as test objects. The laboratory methods that were developed built on work on tissue culture and polioviruses done in the USA, but were more difficult to adapt than had been anticipated. Being able to test materials in volunteers made all the difference in recognising the first limited successes. It was not expected that there would be so many different cold viruses, and having a WHO network greatly helped in sorting them all out. However, the existence of the network did not reveal waves of cold viruses sweeping across the world as had happened in the case of influenza.

Being part of a network made it possible to pass on results and set up collaborations. This was partly because we came to know many of the key players personally, and we shared a commitment to making the WHO programmes work well. On the other hand, when the acute respiratory infections programme was launched this type of relationship did not last. Many of us felt that the long years of rather academic work would be justified by the discovery that some of the 'new' viruses could explain the serious and fatal illnesses in children—three or four million deaths a year throughout the world. But it was not so and once the field studies had shown that 'old' viruses like measles and bacterial infections were at the heart of the problem—and AIDS had also appeared on the scene—it was felt by many that the common cold was not so important.

Infections in the underdeveloped parts of the world are still major causes of disease and death, particularly among children. They reflect the poor social and economic conditions in which they live. But the findings of studies supported by WHO show that with present knowledge the impact of these conditions can be substantially reduced and at low and bearable cost. Furthermore, we can no longer assume that the conditions which damage health are simply a function of low income.

Dr Jacob John, a virologist working in southern India, has pointed out that within India there are some striking contrasts in the health record of states with equally low incomes per head of population. For example Bihar in the north and Kerala in the south have similar incomes, among the lowest in India, but the health statistics of Kerala are far better than those of Bihar, which has a high infant mortality rate. Life expectancy in Kerala approaches that in so-called developed nations. He suggests that the difference is partly due to the better education provided in the south—almost everyone can read and write. In addition the local government supplies basic healthcare and public health throughout the community. The Integrated Management of Childhood Illness scheme developed by WHO includes protocols for handling colds and other respiratory infections as part of basic healthcare, so in principle this could be done widely even when incomes are low.

These examples show the way, but it would be wishful thinking to imagine that it is now possible to upgrade the management of acute respiratory infections throughout the world. In many places health and education get a small share of the limited funds available. Defence or industrial development usually have higher priorities; local corruption can take its toll; and sometimes restructuring charges imposed by the International Monetary Fund or other lending bodies add to the problem.

Nor is it enough to aim at having the right pills available for children or adults suffering from one of a shortlist of diseases. We have to look beyond the treatment and deal with the causes. Pneumonia, for example, kills children who are undernourished or have chronic illnesses. It follows that our approach has to take these other factors into account. When dealing with poor regions we need to implement a complete rural development plan which includes improvements in food supply, diet, hygiene, and living conditions. Medical care is only one component in this plan, and good health the objective.

A balanced healthcare system cannot be imposed effectively from outside. It needs to be supported and 'owned' by local authorities and community leaders who are ready to keep it going. They have to sell it to their people, generate enthusiasm and a will to develop it, and support their staff. Such leaders need to be found and supported over a period of years. It may well be a slow job, particularly at first, but once it can be demonstrated that improvement follows it will give encouragement and hope to others to do the same elsewhere.

CHAPTER 9

A community pest

Folklore surrounding colds must surely exceed in quantity and variety the tales associated with almost any other human experience. Question any number of people and you will receive a similar number of theories on how colds are caught, how to prevent them, and how to cure them. Lack of research in the past and therefore a lack of knowledge has left the field wide open to speculation, and the result has been the profusion of remedies that are still proposed today. Some of these are the result of common-sense ideas but most are based on very shaky foundations. A common element is the tenacity with which these ideas are held, however unlikely.

The trouble is that everyone is an expert on colds, we've all had them so often. They plagued us at school, messed up our social life, and kept us from work. But they can be more than just a nuisance. If we are also prone to some other illness such as asthma, a cold is quite capable of stirring it up badly, so there are wider implications. It is not enough to know that a virus can cause a cold. We need to know who gets colds and how and when. People have been asking questions of this sort over the years, from well before the first viruses were discovered, and they have come up with a lot of answers. Part of our research involved cutting through the folklore to determine what truth might lie behind these contradictory tales.

Travellers' tales and other clues

One story concerns St Kilda and what was ominously called the 'stranger' cold. This tiny, rocky island lies 45 miles to the west of the Outer Hebrides and is Britain's most westerly point. Dr Johnson and James Boswell heard about it on their tour of Scotland in the eighteenth century. Now a sanctuary for thousands of seabirds, it was inhabited until the 1930s, at which point the inhabitants decamped to the mainland. It is hardly surprising that they finally gave up the unequal struggle since boats had difficulty in reaching this rugged isle, and only then when the wind was in the northeast. But visitors did get through now and again and, when they did, it was noticed that colds broke out and affected many of the St Kildans. Some said the plague was brought by the visitors, others blamed the northeast wind.

Early in the twentieth century, when people were searching for a bacterium that caused colds, scientists went to lonely places in the Caribbean and Labrador. They observed outbreaks of colds but no particular throat bacteria to explain them. Then in 1933 there was a striking and well-documented report by two Americans, Paul and Freese, who had studied colds on the island of Spitzbergen. It could not be reached in winter in those days because the Arctic Ocean around it was frozen. Temperatures on land were very low too. At that point colds died out everywhere. Then came the spring, the ice broke up and, within days of the first ship docking, colds broke out and spread far and wide through the community. No incriminating bacteria were found and yet it was clear that an infectious agent had been brought in by the visitors.

But other careful observers thought differently. One of these, Dr Van Loghem in Holland, studied the rise and fall in the number of colds in villages in different parts of the country and observed that they occurred at exactly the same time. He suggested that something in the environment was responsible. In England a Dr Hope-Simpson recorded similar rises and falls in the families of his practice in Gloucestershire and found that they appeared to be closely linked with the outside temperature. He measured this with a thermometer placed under the surface of the soil. These observers and others saw colds as a product of the climate and the seasons, not as the result of a spreading infection.

During the war, a small group of MRC scientists had also been studying the spread of various infections, working from a laboratory at the NIMR in Hampstead. This was the Air Hygiene Unit, first mentioned in Chapter 3. In 1948 its two key workers moved to Salisbury and for several years were housed with the CCU. The two people in question, James Lovelock and Owen Lidwell, continued the pursuit of their separate interests but also contributed to the work on colds both through discussions on the subject and in more practical ways. Their research, by its very nature, had a tendency to converge with ours from time to time.

There were other travellers' tales too. Explorers said that when they arrived back from the wilderness they came down with terrible colds as soon as they reached civilisation. Christopher Andrewes was reminded of this in the early days of the Salisbury unit. Its problem was that it could never produce colds in a complete batch of volunteers when it inoculated them, even with a 'pedigree' virus that had been well studied and carefully stored. About two-thirds

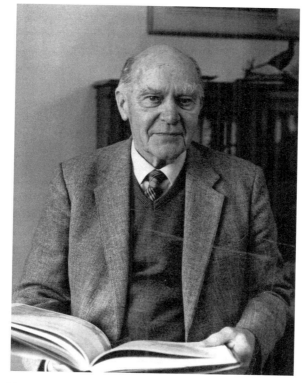

Fig. 9.1 Dr Edgar Hope-Simpson. (From R. E. Hope-Simpson.)

of the volunteers seemed to resist infection. But what would be the effect if they were isolated somewhere for a few months? Perhaps they would all become susceptible.

Seal Island

Andrewes loved novel ideas and anything to do with getting close to nature. Dr Fraser Darling, an expert on the British countryside, told him of an uninhabited island about four miles square, with some houses on it but no electricity or telephone. It lies a mile or so off the west coast of Scotland and is called Eilean nan Ron—Seal Island. It belonged to the Duke of Sutherland and he was willing to lend it for the experiment.

In early July 1950, 12 volunteers, mostly students from Aberdeen, were ferried out to the island by the local boatman. They had a small radio with which to contact the shore and basic food stores, supplied with help from the navy, in spite of strict food rationing. Fishing, it was hoped, and the availability of a few chickens, would help to enliven their meals still further.

The volunteers welcomed the adventure. It was summer, reasonably warm, and the scenery was breathtaking. They did a lot of ringing of nesting seabirds, exploring of caves, observing of seals and basking sharks (the largest of all shark species, reputedly reaching 40 feet), bathing, and fishing. They were enjoying themselves and, apart from a few colds when they arrived, lived there healthily and successfully until mid-September. Then Andrewes and a colleague turned up, thinking they might introduce a cold, but nothing happened. Something more positive was needed.

Six more volunteers were drafted in, inoculated with a pedigree cold in Aberdeen and, as soon as they showed symptoms, shipped over to join the others. Efforts were then made to pass their colds on to the island volunteers. Objects they had touched or sneezed over were given to the islanders to handle. Another group was exposed to the air in a room where cold sufferers had spent time breathing and sneezing. Others lived and ate with some islanders for three days. But no colds were passed on, even when four more infected subjects arrived for another bout of 'maximum exposure'. Then a crofter with a cold came over from the mainland and talked for four hours round a fire with one of the groups. Three of the four developed colds in the next few days. A small success at last.

Andrewes was typically upbeat about the whole exercise. 'Though this laborious experiment failed in its main object it gave us some useful ideas for future work', was his verdict. James Lovelock, who had been helping to run the exercise, said he enjoyed the experience but in retrospect did not think the experiments had been very well devised. One thing the experimenters discovered was that isolation did not make their subjects universally susceptible to colds, which suggested, in spite of the small numbers, that a pedigree virus might not be the same as a 'wild' virus. This was not the sort of research that leads to clear-cut conclusions, but what it did show was that some plausible ideas did not seem to apply and that they should go back to Salisbury, think hard about what had happened, and try to devise some more informative experiments.

Virus spreading is child's play

After Seal Island the Salisbury workers tried to work out the significance of their summer experiments. Local schools were notified that they wanted to invite children with colds to special parties at the unit. Soon they had groups of them, heavy with cold, playing games with volunteers using cards and other objects, even playing 'passing the matchbox' from nose to nose. A number of variations were tried while the children coughed and sneezed their way through each session. In one of these they played games amongst themselves while volunteers sat behind a curtain, to prevent physical contact, but with a fan above it to blow the air towards them. In another, volunteers played with the objects the children had used. Volunteers caught colds following the games sessions with the children, and there were two colds after handling objects which the children had used but some doubt that they were genuine. No colds resulted when the volunteers remained behind a curtain.

During and after the war the Air Hygiene Unit had been influenced by American work on the spread of bacterial infections. This showed that after droplets had been coughed or sneezed out they would dry down to much smaller droplet nuclei. These could carry germs for long distances and then be inhaled. Using early flash photography they had obtained pictures of droplets of all sizes being shot out of the mouth and nose into the air. These seemed an obvious vehicle for the transmission of cold viruses from one person to another. But the experiments with children did not clearly support the idea.

An alternative possibility was suggested via an impressive experiment devised by James Lovelock. He built a rig that trickled a solution of a fluorescent dye out of the nose of one of the laboratory staff. They set it running and then played cards together. After that they turned out the lights and put on a fluorescent lamp. To their amazement they found that the dye had got onto the cards, tables, their fingers, and other parts of the room. This suggested that a cold virus might be moved about on fingers and objects. But the early volunteer experiments showed quite clearly that in order to start a cold it was necessary for the virus to get inside the nose. So what was the method of transmission?

In the next few years little attention was paid to the question of how colds or viruses spread, how colds were caught, or why there were more in winter than in summer. But these questions had not been forgotten. Andrewes would frequently raise the issues over coffee. He favoured the idea that cold viruses lurked in the nose and throat of apparently healthy people and would emerge if some outside conditions activated them. My view was that viruses were spread with some difficulty but were always moving from one person to the next. I also believed that more colds occurred in winter because conditions were then better for viruses to leap from one nose to another.

Unfortunately our level of knowledge at the time made these points purely academic. We could not make further headway or choose between competing

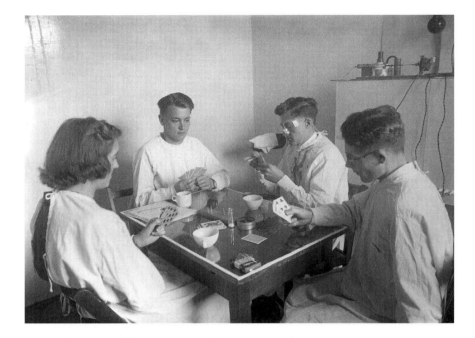

Fig. 9.2 A model experiment on spreading 'virus' by fingers. The individual at the back had a tube running to his nose that slowly leaked a dilute solution of a fluorescent dye while he played cards with his three companions. The one on the right was James Lovelock, who devised the experiment. After the game was over the lights were switched off and an ultraviolet lamp turned on. This showed that the dye was spotted and smeared over each of the players, the table and cards, and even further away. (From the collection of Keith R. Thompson.)

ideas until we had better methods for detecting viruses; and we needed to identify indicators of infection and immunity. Those frustrating early experiments, where we had no choice but to use volunteers, could only take us so far. We would be able to learn far more once we could grow some representative viruses in tissue culture and measure some antibodies.

What happens in families?

In the early post-war years no one really knew how often children and adults got colds. School records showed that some children were kept away from school with colds, but we knew that others continued with their education regardless of such illnesses. And there were no statistics for pre-school children. There were records of general practices, but these told only part of the story since adults and children only went to a doctor if their cold was

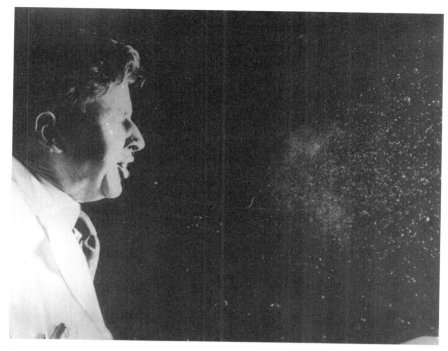

Fig. 9.3 An early flash photograph to demonstrate the cloud of droplets driven out by a sneeze.

particularly bad. For adults that probably meant about one cold in ten. Work records were also incomplete and could be misleading. It was a very uncertain picture, and one which was clearly of concern to the CCU.

Bill Bradley of the Ministry of Health had proposed right from the start that, in addition to carrying out experiments on the cold virus, the CCU should also study the disease and its effects in the community. Dr Tom Somerville, the unit's medical superintendent, decided to throw some light on the subject. The year was 1948 and he began by documenting what was going on in the nearby Wiltshire countryside. It was one of the first studies that the unit carried out. Each week he visited certain families in their homes in villages in the Chalke Valley, a few miles away, travelling in the unit car with matron and the driver, Tom. He would talk to those who were at home and record details of any colds they had suffered.

Somerville, essentially a clinician, was a careful observer ideally suited to a project of this kind. It was simple but serious shoe leather epidemiology. It was also laborious, particularly in winter, but there were compensations. In summer, when the countryside was in full bloom, they would occasionally stop for a picnic. Tom, for his part, made many good friends who he was still meeting in the local pub years later. And when doctor and matron were unable to visit, Tom turned epidemiologist and went round on his own to complete the records.

Months passed and they soon had a formidable collection of statistics—more than sufficient for them to carry out an analysis and see the overall pattern of the illness. The analysis was to be undertaken by Owen Lidwell of the Air Hygiene Unit, an applied mathematician who had already studied outbreaks of illness in school children in London as part of his own research. The results showed that adults living on their own had about one cold a year, while adults in families with schoolchildren averaged over two, and infants five. Schoolchildren had about three. Colds sometimes spread through the family, though the chance of catching one in this way (the secondary attack rate) was only about one in five. These were useful results, and they were confirmed by a further study, using similar methods, which Lidwell carried out on his return to London. He also showed that weather did have an effect on the occurrence of colds.

Hope-Simpson, the GP from Gloucester mentioned earlier, studied the epidemiology of infectious diseases throughout his long life, recording every illness in his practice in Cirencester. Then he and his wife spent their evenings transferring the careful practice notes into epidemiological records. He also recruited some of his patients to keep a daily record of their symptoms on a simple record card. They were remarkably detailed and careful studies in which he tried to take account of all illnesses, whether medical attention was sought or not. Not surprisingly he came up with figures that were much higher than those from the Chalke Valley, calculating that adults had seven colds a year but saw a doctor for only about 5% of these. The differences could be explained by the fact that he was studying a country town and his detailed method of recording would show up periods of mild symptoms that, in different circumstances, might easily be forgotten or overlooked.

While the Salisbury studies were going on, a Dr John Dingle in Cleveland, Ohio was studying local families using a card like Hope-Simpson's. He calculated an average of six respiratory infections a year, and concluded that 'variations in the definition of illnesses…prevent a valid comparison of absolute levels of incidence'. Nevertheless his results and those of Edgar Hope-Simpson have been largely confirmed by others, who have come up with answers in the same range.

The US National Health Survey 1957–61 systematically contacted people, asking them to tell researchers if they had had any health problem in the recent past. The results showed that upper respiratory illnesses occurred throughout the year but increased perhaps threefold in the winter. Even in summer they outnumbered injuries or any other infection. In Cleveland they combined the figures for all the common acute respiratory diseases—colds, rhinitis, bronchitis, laryngitis, etc.—and these accounted for the vast majority of illnesses observed in families. In fact all the figures confirm that colds are the most frequent illness in modern society.

'New' respiratory viruses

Meanwhile, researchers in the USA had demonstrated a range of new techniques for detecting respiratory viruses and, by 1953, the CCU had used John Ender's methods to grow a new virus. Others in the USA were exploiting monkey kidney cultures to grow numerous 'new' viruses (ECHO or Orphan viruses) which they had recently detected. Also in the USA, at the Communicable Diseases Centre, Alex Shelokov showed that influenza virus would grow in monkey kidney cultures and that, even if the cultures looked normal, red cells would stick to virus-infected cells (haemadsorption). This method was applied by Bob Chanock and his team to study croup, pneumonia, and related diseases in children in Washington, DC. And from this work emerged the new group of parainfluenza viruses, of which two members had already been discovered, using eggs.

Hilleman's group in the US Army used human cancer cells, named HeLa after the patient from whom they were grown. These grew easily in the lab and were readily infected and killed by polioviruses. It turned out that they were also killed by adenoviruses, related to those grown from children's tonsils, though these were found in samples taken from the throats of servicemen with feverish sore throats and bronchitis.

Chanock's group used similar cultures to show that yet another 'new' virus—respiratory syncytial virus—caused most cases of bronchiolitis in infants, a respiratory disease that can be fatal.

The middle of the 1950s saw a remarkably successful rush to grow viruses from children in hospital using the novel tissue cultures. But there was very little to relate about the growth of viruses from older children or adults in the community suffering from common colds. Two reports from the USA in 1957 claimed that a virus—called JH or 2060—had been grown from a few adults with colds.

Viruses in the community

This was the background to common cold research when I reached the unit in 1957. Although remote physically from other workers in the field, we were kept informed through monthly journals and occasional letters and reports from abroad. And these told us that many competent people were forging ahead in this work. In what way could we contribute most effectively to this pattern of research? I knew that we had in our favour a laboratory team with years of hard-won experience and the unique volunteer scheme. It was simply a question of how we could best apply these resources. We decided that we would identify the things that we could do well, then choose something from among those that others were not doing and work very hard at it. If we combined different parts of the new techniques with some bright ideas of our own we could gradually develop a new technique for growing a cold virus. And we had the advantage of being able to use our volunteers to test the results. Our work met with some success and, by 1960, we had methods which enabled us to detect rhinoviruses, but only in about one in four people with colds.

The discovery of respiratory viruses had naturally led curious minds around the world to wonder if they accounted for all common colds and related diseases. By the early 1960s some patterns were emerging. Adenoviruses types 1, 2, and 5 were usually found in the throats of small children, frequently without causing them any discomfort though occasionally they had colds or sore throats. Types 3, 4, 7, and 21 occurred more typically in older children as well as in servicemen during training, causing fever and a sore throat, bronchitis or, occasionally, conjunctivitis. Parainfluenza viruses caused chest infections such as croup and pneumonia. RSV caused acute bronchiolitis in infants but did not seem to be present in ordinary colds.

Much of this information came from the USA, and we wondered to what extent these viruses were present in community illnesses in Britain. Representatives of the parainfluenza viruses were given to Salisbury volunteers and produced common cold-like diseases, but nothing more serious. Possibly such viruses were quite common in our community, causing our volunteers to become partly immune. When we checked specimens from various patients, the boys of Epsom College, our volunteers, and staff, we found mainly rhinoviruses. It was all rather confusing.

We needed to look more closely at what was going on outside the unit and decided to set up a nationwide study of all these respiratory viruses. Help was sought from virus workers in the Public Health Laboratory Service and the clinicians they worked with. Sympathetic clinicians were also contacted in paediatric departments, general practice, and so on, and asked to study typical patients at regular intervals. All agreed to cooperate in the project, even though we were adding considerably to their normal workload; and it is a tribute to their dedication that the whole scheme ultimately worked so well.

We began by running a 'mini-course' at the CCU, advising them on how the samples were to be collected and tested. This helped the virologists to get to know each other and made collaboration much easier.

Months later the work of these helpful clinicians had produced numerous blue record cards piled high on a bench in Salisbury, awaiting analysis. It was to be a laborious task, conducted with paper and pencil—in the early 1960s we had no computers—but well worth the effort. The results gave us an insight into the prevalence of virus strains in the community and showed that all the different groups of viruses were circulating. Almost any virus could be found in any disease, from colds at the top of the airways to bronchitis and pneumonia at the bottom. But each virus, or group of viruses, tended to attack particular areas more frequently or more severely, and first-time infections in children were usually more severe than re-infections in later life. And the fact that these viruses were much less likely to be found in healthy members of the patients' families provided strong evidence that they caused the diseases.

It must be admitted that the number of patients was relatively small and the sampling methods were not perfect, and so some investigators thought the whole study should be conducted again more rigorously. This was done but with similar results. Nevertheless it was clear that our set-up was not best suited to large-scale field research.

Although we now knew that rhinoviruses were causing colds in the community, we still could not detect a virus of any sort in most people with colds. We had to find better methods of detection. This took some time, but eventually we were successful in establishing culture methods for growing rhinoviruses and other, as yet unknown, viruses. And this led to our discovery of coronaviruses, mentioned earlier. Since then these have been largely supplanted by molecular methods.

Workers in the USA also joined in the hunt for these newly discovered viruses in their communities. For example the 'Virus Watch' programmes, first in New York City and later in Seattle, looked particularly for rhinoviruses in families living at home. Others studied colds in offices and amongst servicemen and students. In all cases more rhinoviruses were found than any other virus, but in only a quarter to a third of all cases. It was a reasonable guess that rhinoviruses were the most important cause of colds. But how could one prove this when viruses could still not be detected in the majority of cases?

How colds spread

One day I was preparing a chapter for a book on common colds and reading what medical textbooks said about how colds spread. They wrote that it was by coughing and sneezing out saliva. But this was all guesswork—there was not one reference to any proper experiments on the subject. I knew we could do better than that. We had our human guinea pigs, and with their assistance we would carry out some meaningful research.

Our inability to handle rhinoviruses easily in the early 1960s drove us into looking for an alternative, which would cause typical colds like a rhinovirus but could be more readily manipulated. It was a man called Coe, a serviceman in California, who provided us with the first strain of just such a virus. Although it came from the nose it was found to be neutralised by serum against a coxsackie virus type 21 which, like other coxsackie viruses, was originally found in the gut. Thus it was related to the poliovirus family, but behaved like a rhinovirus.

Peggy Pereira sent us a British strain which she had isolated and we showed that it caused typical colds in our volunteers if given as nose-drops. The advantage from our point of view was that few, if any, of our volunteers had been infected by this virus in the past and so did not have the appropriate antibodies. As a result most of them developed colds. Virus could be detected by inoculating nasal secretions into suitable tissue cultures; and antibodies in the blood could be measured by a simple haemagglutination inhibition test, rather like the standard influenza test.

We needed a research worker to begin the study, someone with an interest in the subject and the necessary background knowledge. We were fortunate to find such a person in the form of Dr Frank Buckland. A man of wide interests, he was brought up on a large country estate in Lincolnshire where he had developed a life-long interest in country sports, particularly fly-fishing. Medical school led to the army where he became interested in pathology and, particularly, bacteriology; and it was in this subject that he began to do research. After the war he helped to establish the Microbiological Research Establishment at Porton Down, near Salisbury, eventually becoming deputy director. During the Suez Crisis he was called away to serve as brigadier in charge of the army medical laboratories. When he returned he was due to be demobilised, and retired.

Buckland's dream had always been that he would retire to a country house and indulge in his love of gardening, but still maintain an interest in medical research. The first half of his dream was satisfied when he bought a house with a large garden at Coombe Bissett, a couple of miles away from the CCU. And almost immediately after his arrival there he heard about our need for a specialist research worker. An unusual and kindly man, he had a reputation for creating a happy atmosphere wherever he worked; and his wide research experience made him an ideal candidate for the role we had in mind. The formalities of his appointment were soon completed and he came to work as an assistant researcher at the unit, a few minutes drive from his home.

The Microbiological Research Establishment had extensive laboratories and a large staff whose job was to develop methods of defending the country against biological weapons being assembled in the USSR. It was thought that pathogenic bacteria might be delivered by spraying cultures to form clouds that would drift over cities. To analyse what might happen they studied clouds of harmless organisms and then measured their concentration and their fate when inhaled. Buckland, with his contacts there, was able to borrow appropriate sampling equipment and supplies of harmless bacteria from the Microbiological Research Establishment. We also drew on our links with the MRC bioengineers to ask them to develop a small aerosol spray (like a scent spray) that would produce droplets of the same size and quantity as those expelled by a human sneeze.

We wanted to work out how secretions were driven out of the mouth and nose in coughs and sneezes, and to do this we needed a suitable tracer. James Lovelock was the man to help here, and so we asked him to come down and talk with us about the problem. Perhaps we could use the fluorescent dye he had employed. He sat down in the lab, listened to our story and then, for about an hour, produced a torrent of suggestions for likely and unlikely techniques.

Buckland kept notes of these but by the end was in despair. How could we possibly find time to work our way through all these? I assured him that we would not even try. We would simply sift through all the ideas produced by Lovelock's brain-storming and pick the one that best suited our needs. The possibility of using bacterial spores was the one that appealed most. So Buckland raised a stock of spores from Porton and we were able to move straight into productive experimentation.

Right on the nose

The Air Hygiene Unit had used the level of mouth bacteria in the air as an indicator of how likely the mouth was to be carrying cold germs, but we were more interested in the nose. This was because our research suggested that cold viruses were mainly present in the nose and not the mouth. It also appeared that viruses had to get back into the nose in order to start an infection. This was where we planned to focus our attention (See Fig. 9.3).

Research had shown that very small particles, under 5 µm (a µm, or micrometre, is 10^{-6} metres) in diameter, were the most numerous in the air after a sneeze. Because of their lightness such particles could remain

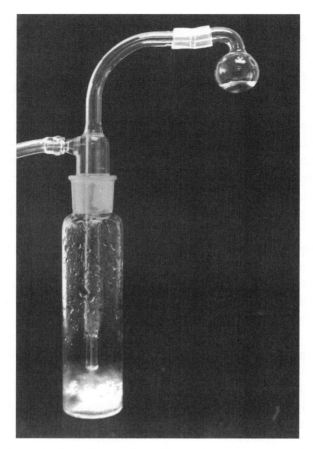

Fig. 9.4 The Porton impinger for sampling airborne viruses or bacteria. Those carried by particles likely to be trapped in the nose were collected in the small sphere. Those on smaller particles likely to land in the lower airways were collected in the cylinder. A vacuum pump was attached to the small tube on the left and air was sucked through the device at the rate of normal breathing. The fluids were removed and tested for the amount of virus they contained. (© Barry Dowsett, CAMR, Porton Down.)

suspended for long periods and be carried considerable distances, making them of particular interest in biological warfare. However, these would not be trapped by mucus in the nose but would carry infection down the lower airways into the lungs. We were not interested in these at this stage. Fortunately a sneeze also produces larger particles, varying between 5 μm and 20 μm. These settle out quite slowly and, if inhaled, will stick in the nose.

The Microbiological Research Establishment had developed a simple glass device called the Porton impinger, through which air could be sucked. This would then separate the particles, collecting the larger ones in a small sphere and all the small ones in fluid in a large glass cylinder. And it was these we used in our attempts to analyse a sneeze. First we placed a drop of spore suspension in the nose of each subject. Then, with their heads inside a large plastic bag, they tickled their noses with a little probe until they sneezed. We sucked the air out through an impinger to find what was present of the two classes of particles, and washed the inside surface of the bag to discover what had come out as large blobs. The latter could get onto hands and surfaces but could not be inhaled.

It transpired, as one would expect, that the largest amount of what was expelled in a sneeze or snort was in the form of large blobs. The impinger samples showed a few spores in the fine droplets but far more of them in the 5–20 µm particles. These dropped only gradually to the floor and would be caught in the nose if they were breathed in. This suggested that these medium-sized droplets were the most likely to contain enough virus and to transmit an infection.

Similar experiments were carried out on volunteers with colds due to Coe virus. These showed that there was rarely any virus in the smallest droplets, but measurable amounts in the 5–20 µm fraction and more still on the walls of the bag. This was very similar to what we had found with the tracer spores. But would droplets like these actually transmit infection? To avoid the complications and difficulties of one volunteer infecting another we devised a rather unusual test.

The wardrobe experiment

Among the items of furniture in daily use in the unit were some red pine wardrobes, kindly left behind by our American friends. They served us well, providing much-needed hanging space, but now we had a rather different use in mind for one of them.

First we took a chair, placed it inside, and persuaded a volunteer to sit on it. It was a fairly tight squeeze, but that was one of its advantages—we did not want any excess space. A hole was cut in one of the side walls alongside the subject's head so the mouth of an impinger could be inserted to sample the air he or she was breathing. Loosening the top of the wardrobe then enabled us to insert our hand-spray, filled with virus suspension, and use it to deliver an artificial sneeze in the direction of the subject's head and face. It was all very simple, and very effective.

One by one, groups of subjects were exposed to infection in this way and then observed for the next five days, as was customary. The virus recovered from the sampler indicated how much virus they had breathed in and the results of the virus tests on their nose and blood showed whether they had been infected.

The results were clear: volunteers who inhaled one or more infectious virus particles were infected provided they were not immune. So it was plausible to conclude that people sneezed out virus in droplets that others could inhale and become infected with. And since everyone breathes air at about 10 litres per minute throughout the day, a small amount of infectious material in the air would be enough to pass virus from one person to another.

Our wardrobe experiment caused some amusement but it was scientifically sound. And it worked: it confirmed our suppositions concerning transmission of cold viruses and provided a firm foundation on which to develop further research projects.

American workers had been doing similar but independent work using the Coe virus. They were able to show that the virus could spread from one end of a hut to the other even though volunteers with colds were separated by a double-wire mesh screen from those who were healthy. This ensured that, although droplets could pass through, fingers and objects could not. In another experiment volunteers inhaled an aerosol consisting of fine droplets of a virus preparation and became infected. But the area attacked was down the bronchial tree and not just the nose—as predicted.

From the Arctic to the Kalahari

Stories of cold epidemics in Spitzbergen suggested that these coincided with the arrival of warm spring weather. My belief was that colds and similar illnesses were particular problems for those who lived in temperate climates with cold seasons. However, conversations with people from the tropics, and the evidence of my own eyes during occasional visits, made me realise that runny noses and coughs were not confined to places like Britain—they occurred in hot countries too. It was not practical to go travelling and collect samples from people with respiratory symptoms of this sort, but we could do what had been done with other virus infections, such as poliomyelitis, and test blood sera from people living in these countries.

We now had tests for antibodies and knew that most individuals developed such antibodies after they were infected. So we could test the sera and discover whether the viruses we had found in Britain were infecting and possibly causing illness in other parts of the world. A number of scientists had made collections of sera and were willing to send us small samples from what was left in their refrigerators. Fortunately sera are quite stable and still retain the antibodies years after they have been collected.

Serological surveys like this were conducted for a number of years and we quickly learned some important facts. In the first place, antibodies against a selection of respiratory viruses were common in sera collected in widely separated parts of the world. It looked as though the viruses we had grown were not peculiar to our region but were part of a general health problem. Certain ones, like the parainfluenza and respiratory syncytial virus, infected in the first few years of life. Some collections of sera suggested that antibodies become more common in people as they pass from childhood into adulthood, suggesting that people infected with a series of viruses gradually build up immunity against them one by one.

Sera from remote communities such as Inuit in the Arctic would have relatively few antibodies, we thought, because the viruses would not reach them very often. However, we found that their antibody pattern was very much like those in towns elsewhere in the world, and the same applied to Bushmen of the Kalahari Desert in their very different sort of isolation. On talking to those who knew these areas we discovered that, in the second half of the twentieth century, these peoples were not totally cut off. There were a few visitors to Arctic settlements throughout the year, and the Bushmen often lived on the fringe of the desert for part of the year, or visited villages and settlements to trade and so on. It seemed that such contacts were enough to enable the viruses to spread into their society from the outside world.

Tristan da Cunha

One place alone provided us with sera which were genuinely lacking in antibodies against these viruses. A research institute in South Africa had collected sera from the islanders of Tristan da Cunha to test for antibodies against poliovirus and we found that these sera had antibodies against relatively few of our panel of respiratory viruses. It was clear that there must be some connection between the island's remoteness and such low levels of antibodies. Ships called only a few times a year to pick up water during long voyages through the southern oceans. Otherwise visits tended to be confined to those periods when the weather was favourable for fishing and for small boats delivering supplies or taking off passengers. The ships came mostly from South Africa and some from South America. A few cruise-ships also passed by.

A British possession, the island functioned as a diminutive colony with an administrator, doctor, and school. The population consisted of some 300 people, the descendants of British soldiers, stationed there while Napoleon was being held on the island of St Helena, or of settlers from the crews of old whaling ships. They lived in simple cottages and kept themselves by farming and fishing, and had a small crayfish cannery with which they earned cash by exporting, mainly to South Africa. But, for most of the time, they were isolated from contact with strangers. Nevertheless it was said that epidemics of colds sometimes spread around the island after a boat's visit. This all seemed quite logical, and we concluded that extreme isolation was needed to prevent cold viruses reaching a community.

Studying what was happening in the rest of the world gave us the broad view that we needed, and helped to put our experiments on volunteers into perspective. Of course we already had well-established overseas contacts through WHO, but financial restraints would normally put places like Tristan da Cunha well outside our range. However, fate was to provide us with further opportunities for making contact with the people of this remote South Atlantic island. Like many others of its kind, it is in fact the tip of a volcano. And in 1961 it erupted.

Suddenly this peaceful and remote community, virtually unknown to the outside world, found itself on the front page of every newspaper. Lava and ash swept down the mountainside and eventually into the village, forcing the evacuation of the inhabitants. They took a few personal belongings and sailed off to a world most of them had never seen. First stop was Cape Town, but apartheid was then in full force and they were not welcome. Britain accepted responsibility and arranged for them to be housed in empty service accommodation in the south of England. They were within easy reach of Salisbury.

Although they had stopped only briefly in South Africa some of them had caught colds and these spread throughout the community on the voyage to Europe. It was generally agreed that the colds were unusually severe and some elderly islanders had serious chest complaints. They were in urgent need of medical attention. They also displayed a number of characteristics, such as allergies and congenital abnormalities, that were of interest to biological and medical research. However, I am glad to say that respect for their sensibilities as well as concern for their well-being prevented a wholesale rush of medics in their direction. It was agreed that it would be unpleasant for them and probably counterproductive if a range of investigators descended on them as they settled in.

A committee was formed and it was agreed that we would minimise the amount of contact with outsiders and the number of samples collected. This

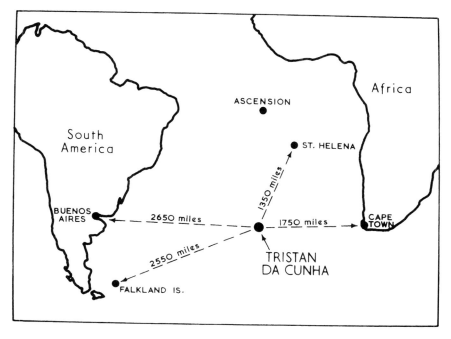

Fig. 9.5 One of the world's remotest islands, Tristan da Cunha in the South Atlantic.

meant that we could have blood samples to test for antibodies but could not meet or talk to islanders or collect samples for virus tests. Medical attention would be provided by their own doctor. A few specialist interviewers would make contact but all studies would be agreed with them and channelled through the people they knew.

Even this may sound as if they were being imposed upon, but in fact it worked well for most of those concerned. We had no clinical records of their illnesses or specimens for virus isolation but we were given samples of their sera. These showed that they had been infected with viruses prevalent in Britain but absent from their island. We could not sort out which infection had caused which disease but it was clear that, as far as their resistance was concerned, they had come into England with very little natural immunity and, rather like a baby just born into the world, had suffered badly from the viruses they were meeting for the first time.

Our strange culture was not to their liking and they were clearly longing to return to their island home. When the eruption had died down, an advance party returned to make essential repairs and ensure that there was somewhere decent for them to live. In 1963 almost all of them decided to return and take up their lives on Tristan again.

We wondered whether the old pattern of colds would be re-established and whether we would be able to document what happened. The research committee helped in this and it was arranged that the island medical officer would make it his research project: he would record the coming and going of ships, the occurrence of colds in all the families, and some clinical features of the outbreaks. He used simple cards to record the symptoms and kept the study going meticulously. As the years passed it was fascinating to see a return to the old pattern that had existed before the eruption. Waves of colds started to appear, usually within days of a ship calling, especially when coming from Cape town; ships coming from other ports were at sea so long that any colds on board when they started had died out before they reached Tristan. Sometimes the first case could be traced back to an islander who had gone aboard a ship, or to a person from the ship who had come ashore with a cold. But there were occasions when the virus must have been brought ashore by someone without symptoms.

Symptoms and the way the illness spread were not the same on each occasion and so we surmised that more than one type of cold virus was responsible. But we had no specimens with which to prove it. Later on a severe outbreak of influenza almost brought normal life on Tristan to a halt. Our tests on a few serum specimens showed that it was an outbreak of influenza A, probably the same type that was epidemic around the world at the time.

This natural experiment proved conclusively that the people who were on the island had normal susceptibility to infection and were not naturally immune. The unusual and infrequent cold epidemics were simply due to the very limited contact they had with the outside world.

Colds in the freezer

This experience encouraged us to look around for other remote colonies. And what could be more remote than the South Pole? As it happened, the British Antarctic Survey always had a medically qualified person in each group of research workers spending the winter at any of their Antarctic bases. Being cut off completely for about six months each year made it essential to have someone on hand to deal with medical emergencies. Ironically this period, which of course was the winter, was also the time when there was hardly ever any illness about and therefore very little for a young medic to do. An ideal antidote for boredom and a better use of resources was to use this opportunity for a research project, preferably one for which the unique environment was

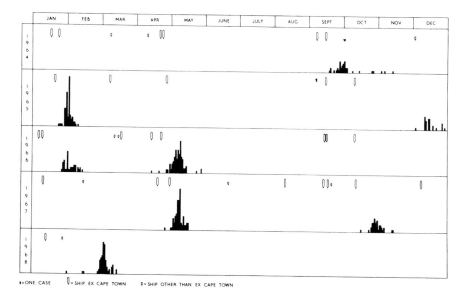

Fig. 9.6 The number of colds suffered by the island's population after they returned from Britain. Waves of colds occurred usually just after a ship called and especially if it came from South Africa, a relatively short voyage. (From Cliff *et al. Island Epidemics*, 2000.)

particularly suited. Usually this involved matters of human physiology and the effects of the extreme conditions. The situation seemed to be tailor-made for the sort of research we had in mind.

We knew that respiratory infections did occur in the region, and there were classical explorers' tales of how a wave of colds would go round a base when a new group arrived in the spring. There were also stories of how colds would appear and spread, sometimes after a long period of isolation, perhaps when a container of clothing was opened. It was a good opportunity to try and document some of these stories. It might also be possible to introduce viruses we had studied in England, and to measure how they spread and what effects they produced in these very crowded conditions. At the CCU people had tried to get viruses to spread from one volunteer to another but very little happened; perhaps because of the sort of accommodation we used. On the other hand, some stories suggested that when a cold got into one of the base huts down south it usually spread quite freely.

One particular member of the MRC staff, Dr Otto Edholm, who headed the Human Physiology Unit, had good contacts with the British Antarctic Survey and frequently arranged research projects with them. He knew about the stories of colds in Antarctica. He also knew that I was interested and on one occasion offered to arrange for me to visit one of their bases so that I could see the situation for myself. I was sorely tempted, having previously tried to join an expedition there soon after I qualified. However, it meant a long sea voyage and leaving the department, volunteers, patients, wife, and family for several months. I felt it would be irresponsible and, reluctantly, declined. But the project went ahead—Edholm found two young medics, already selected to go south, who were interested in doing work on virus infections and colds. I had to be content with observing proceedings from a distance of some ten thousand miles.

Drs Mike Holmes and Terry Allen were the ones who had taken an interest in the project. Their first step was to come to the unit for a period of training and experience in the clinical and laboratory study of colds and to read up on the literature. Preliminary work was then begun and a protocol developed. Mike Holmes' plan was to release an influenza virus and a cold virus (coxsackievirus A21) and see what happened. But first we needed to settle whether the research workers were willing to be human guinea pigs, and to sort out the practical problems of preparing, storing, and transporting samples to a centrally heated hut surrounded by the equivalent of a deep freeze cabinet. Both matters were resolved satisfactorily and the experiment began. But the results were not very startling. Yes, the volunteers did become infected, but the illnesses were mild and like those seen in the UK. One other thing was clear—the laboratory procedures needed to be improved.

Mike Holmes used the next Antarctic season to do laboratory work at Salisbury, but then wanted to experience another winter of Antarctic life and take his experiments further. This time he would wait until isolation was established before releasing the HGP strain of rhinovirus. Of the 17 people wintering in the very congested hut, 9 were to be infected. Blood specimens would then be collected and clinical records prepared in the usual way. Nasal specimens were to be mixed with a buffered solution that he had developed with a visiting French worker and unit staff, and the samples brought back to Salisbury for virological testing.

Somehow Holmes persuaded his colleagues to cooperate and, in spite of the extreme conditions and the problems of refrigeration and transport, completed virus testing. The major finding was that the virus successfully infected a number of subjects, causing colds much like those seen in Britain. He also carefully studied the effects of the same virus on a comparison group of volunteers in Salisbury. His conclusion was that the colds seemed to be worse in Antarctica, and the virus grew more vigorously in the nose—though it was hard to be sure about the latter. What he did find, though, was that the amount of antibody in the nasal secretions gradually declined during the period of isolation, reducing resistance. This fits with explorers' claims that they have worse colds when they first leave isolation.

Terry Allen studied outbreaks of colds in British Antarctic Survey bases in 1970 and showed that colds died out during isolation and returned within a few days of a ship's arrival. Similarly, men had colds within a few days of boarding a ship for the journey home. Such colds were rather worse than colds that occurred on base. Again this confirmed the old explorers' stories and the records from Tristan da Cunha.

I would like to have studied isolated communities in more detail. Quite probably a few very remote tribes, such as those in the Amazon rain forest, have had similar experiences, but I had no opportunity to check this out.

Our work in this field had one very happy sequel. John Mackenzie, a student at the University of Edinburgh, visited the laboratory during the summer vacation when some of this work was going on. He wanted the experience and could also take the opportunity of visiting relatives who lived in the vicinity of the unit. It seems that this brief contact with the staff and the projects current at the time fired his interest in influenza and other viruses. Since then he has pursued a successful academic career in Australia, with posts in Perth and Brisbane, eventually becoming a professor with a department of his own.

The unit was also a source of further inspiration for at least one novel exercise subsequently introduced into Mackenzie's medical virology teaching programme. Students are asked to imagine a mythical island in the South Pacific called Raraponga! It is extremely isolated, has a small weather station, and a volcano which suddenly erupts. The inhabitants have to be evacuated to Sydney. What, the students are asked, do they think would be the effect on the viral disease burden of the evacuees, and how should the authorities deal with the situation?

Apparently it is still a very popular exercise with the students.

Fingers and fomites

Meanwhile, James Lovelock was much impressed by his demonstration that nasal secretion could spread widely around a person with a cold. And there were others who thought that colds might be spread in this way. One group in Charlottesville, Virginia took this very seriously and worked on the subject for some years. They were able to show that rhinovirus could be present on fingers and might remain for several hours, disappearing or becoming non-infectious quite slowly. They also demonstrated that virus could survive on household objects and be transferred from skin to skin on contact. A film of a local Sunday school class showed that well brought up American children and adults frequently picked at their noses and rubbed their fingers in their eyes. So if a person picked up a virus, from a surface in a room for example, they might, in this way, inadvertently transfer it to a point on the body where it could gain access. All this implied that virus could be passed by contact from a cold sufferer to a healthy individual. The question was how often did this happen?

The answer, the researchers decided, might be found if they could devise an effective form of nasal tissue that would inactivate viruses and provide a useful form of cold prevention. Controlled trials were set up amongst local families in which half used these medicated wipes and the other half a similar but un-medicated tissue. The families were monitored both clinically and virologically, and the study lasted for two winter seasons. The results showed very little difference between the number of colds caught in the two groups of families, although there may have been a marginal reduction in the number of colds caused by rhinoviruses.

Sylvia Reed, one of our researchers, took on the task of re-examining this problem. Born and brought up in the Midlands, Sylvia studied medicine at Cambridge where she became interested in viruses. Clinical work followed in the Department of Bacteriology at the London Hospital in Whitechapel. She was then able to spend a year at the new MRC virology unit in Glasgow, a very active research centre, which was making important advances in the fundamental biology of viruses. And it was there that she became involved in a project studying why certain adenoviruses produce tumours in animals but did not seem to do so in humans. This led to a desire to look at other forms of virus growth and, in particular, the study of viruses growing in human volunteers and in organ cultures of human airway cells. She knew of our work in Salisbury and, on hearing of our vacancy, took the opportunity of joining us.

Sylvia Reed studied the transfer of infection to and from volunteers as thoroughly and quantitatively as she could, with results that, in some respects, confirmed those of the Americans. Volunteers with colds had virus on their hands and on the cups and other utensils used in their flats. However, the amounts were small and declined steadily with time, and it was difficult to effect any further contamination of fingers from these items. Even transfer of virus from a contaminated finger was not very efficient. Tests on the fingers of 18 volunteers, whose partners were at the peak of a typical rhinovirus cold, did not recover a single virus.

Some years earlier we had shown that virus in a swab dabbed onto the inside of the nose or eye would infect, but Reed thought it unlikely that, in a normal home environment, anyone would have enough virus on a finger to be able to infect themselves. But we could not be absolutely certain that this could not happen. In some circumstances, say a mother nursing or washing a baby with a cold, it may be more likely than an airborne infection.

An American, Elliott Dick of the University of Minnesota, was intrigued by this question of how colds spread. When he learned of Mike Holmes' 'Hut' experiment he decided to duplicate the situation in his department and see if this would give him some answers. He selected non-immune volunteers and infected half their number with a known rhinovirus. Those that caught colds were then cooped up in a small room with the uninfected volunteers and told to play cards with them for several hours. Many of the latter developed colds. The viruses were carefully monitored and he was now sure that he could make colds spread whenever he wanted. He also established, as we had with the children in Salisbury, that playing with cards previously used by people with colds was not enough—the volunteers had to be in the room together.

In one quite bizarre experiment he fitted volunteers with large plastic collars which allowed them to touch cards, table, and fingers but prevented them from touching their faces. The same method is used to prevent a dog from scratching a diseased ear. This suggested that any spread of virus must be through the air. But then he somewhat contradicted this assumption by describing another experiment in which the spread seemed to have been prevented by treating the volunteers' fingers with an antiviral material. So the matter is not completely resolved—a familiar situation in science.

I believe the unit made a useful contribution to the international search for an answer to the question of how colds are spread. But I have to admit that the evidence so far is conflicting. It is true that a mother caring for a baby with a cold may catch the virus by getting it on her fingers. Nevertheless, it is my belief that colds are hardly ever transferred by hand or finger contact.

CHAPTER 10

Looking into the mind

'History is more or less bunk', claimed Henry Ford, and maybe it is. Certainly, if we accept that it is written by the winners, then we must expect some distortion. But here we talk of politics. Other accounts going back over the centuries may be considered more reliable—and, perhaps, more inspiring. Philosophical writings from ancient Greece and onwards continue to guide our thoughts and inform our actions. And amongst these treasures of ancient learning there is much about man's attempts to understand the workings of the human body, as we discovered in Chapter 1. But what about those obscure areas where the mind plays its part?

René Descartes, the French philosopher and mathematician living in the first half of the seventeenth century, provides us with an example of how ideas can reach out to us over the passage of time. He thought deeply about the subjective nature of the senses, and from this derived his famous dictum: *Cogito, ergo sum*—I think, therefore I am. He believed that we consist essentially of two parts: body and mind. But long before that, some 16 centuries earlier, the Roman poet and satirist, Juvenal, made clear that he, too, understood the importance of this relationship with his recommendation *orandum est ut sit mens sana in corpore sano*—you should pray to have a sound mind in a sound body. And, in this third millennium, we accept the idea when we talk of a healthy mind in a healthy body.

Other ancient sources, such as the Bible, seem to suggest that different parts of our being are interdependent. Greek physicians certainly thought so and looked at health and disease in a holistic or all-inclusive way. Yet it was not until the twentieth century that there was any serious attempt to investigate the influences of the mind over the body in matters of health.

We at the CCU had no plans to enter this field. However, our interest in possible drug treatment of colds led us inexorably towards a deeper involvement, and in the end we found ourselves doing a major study in conjunction with colleagues in the USA. The results have attracted wide interest.

Mind over body

For much of the time it matters little whether we think of mind and body as separate or as parts of a single whole, but at the unit we came to learn that it is important in an illness—even one as ordinary as a common cold. Anecdotal evidence suggested that there might be a link but I did not take this possibility very seriously—not at first, that is—until an experiment 'went wrong' or rather, it gave an unforeseen result. This led to a fascinating area of research in which we accumulated solid scientific evidence that there is a relationship between mind and body that affects our susceptibility to an infectious disease and ability to overcome it. The research continues to this day.

Medical opinion has fluctuated in its response to this idea over the years. It was not until the nineteenth and twentieth centuries that pathology was first studied as a science, and it changed the way doctors treated their patients. For example, physicians recognised that some people felt tired and depressed, gained weight, and had a dry skin because their thyroid gland was not producing its hormone. Once they replaced the thyroid hormone all was well: the abnormal signs and unpleasant feelings disappeared. Something similar happened with infections. Feverish people were probably infected. The remedy was to find the invading bacterium and inject the new antibiotic that would kill it. The temperature fell, delirium and distress disappeared, and the person was cured.

Many patients might suffer serious disturbances of their emotions and thinking, which would alter their behaviour but were not the result of any diagnosed medical condition and did not seem to affect the working of their bodies. These patients were classified together as having mental illnesses because the problem seemed to be in their thinking and feeling rather than in the tissues of their bodies.

But it became clear that there were some conditions in which the cause was not so simple. For instance, coronary thrombosis—clotting of blood in the coronary arteries supplying the heart—was a frequent cause of heart attack, and was brought on by several factors in a person's life such as diet, smoking, and lack of exercise. But personality was also important: pushy A-type people were more at risk. And stress can affect the amount of clotting factors in the blood.

Some doctors felt that the effect of the mental state in certain illnesses was so important that they should be classified together in a separate group and called psychosomatic (or mind–body) diseases. A professor of medicine at New York Hospital, Dr Wolff, had a patient called Tom who, as a result of an old injury, had a hole through which the lining of his stomach could be observed. This became reddened if he was upset, suggesting a connection between emotion and symptoms such as indigestion. And so Dr Wolff's students learned that if a patient had indigestion it was important to enquire about his state of mind as well as what went into his stomach. There were many examples of this sort of thing.

One of the sad facts about the application of what has been called 'the body–mind dichotomy' is that body-based diseases were thought of as real while those in the mind were not. Patients might be told by friends or medical advisers that their illness is 'all in the mind', implying that it was not a real problem and would go away if they 'pulled themselves together'. Those who have met or known of someone with a major depressive illness, such as Winston Churchill and his 'black dog', will realise that mental illness is a genuine and serious affliction which does not recover in response to exhortations. Modern research shows that in such cases the brain and nervous system are not working normally. Lesser degrees of mental disturbance show no obvious physical effects but can affect general health along with other factors. In such cases it is hard to tell what each is doing or even if there is a mental component involved.

Avoiding prejudice

We recognised from the start that there were no objective clinical laboratory tests to show that a person had a cold—unlike, say, anaemia where a blood test measures quantitatively whether the problem is there and, if so, how great it is. Instead we had to ask our volunteers whether they had a sore throat, headache, or any other signs of a cold. This was a perfectly acceptable approach, provided we could have confidence in the truth of their responses. When conducting these trials we always gave some participants a placebo—an inactive material—while others had active virus or drug. The problem was that individuals would tend to describe their symptoms in line with what they thought had happened in the experiment—for example, whether they had been given virus or salt water.

But these quite natural reactions were not confined to the volunteers. Human nature also played its part in the response of the observing doctors, and their views would be coloured by what they foresaw as the likely results. As strict scientists they would try to keep their enthusiasm under control and downplay anything they were told. Their cautious approach would therefore be in direct conflict with our keen volunteers who wanted to help science by talking about their cold symptoms in glowing terms. In other words, both were putting their own 'spin' on the observations. We had to eliminate this mental factor.

Our solution was to ensure that neither the observer nor the subject had any way of knowing what had been administered. The over-enthusiastic volunteer would be wary of claiming, 'I think I've got a definite scratchiness in my throat this morning, doctor', if he might be told after the trial that he had been given salt solution and no virus. The observer's views would also receive no stimulus in either direction. This so-called double-blind, placebo-controlled trial proved to be an effective method, introducing a more rigid discipline into our procedures and giving us much greater confidence in the accuracy of our results. We also introduced a very simple and objective method of measuring how much the nose ran. Each volunteer collected, in plastic bags, the handkerchiefs used over a given period, which were then weighed. The dry weight was already known and the difference between the two represented the weight of fluid that had run from the nose.

Interestingly I noticed that observer bias was not restricted to clinical observations. We used to read the haemagglutination tests by eye—looking at the red cells settling to the bottom of a test tube and judging whether the pattern meant agglutination or not. What we wanted to see was less agglutination in those tubes where we expected interference, and sure enough, that was the result. But if someone mixed up the tubes and relabelled them, so that the observer did not know what to expect in any particular tube, then the effect was even more noticeable. It was clear that in our desire not to be biased we

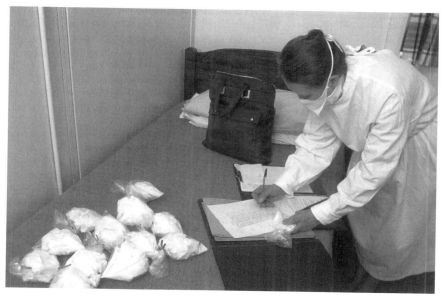

Fig. 10.1 Matron counting out the volunteers' tissues used in 24 hours at the height of a cold. There were five tissues in each bag and they were later weighed in the laboratory to work out the weight of nasal secretions produced, an objective measure of the response to a virus.

would over-compensate, recording results higher than the true ones and so falsely reducing the evidence for interference.

Psychology also plays its part in the way subjects respond to treatment. Many research workers and doctors have observed and documented improvements in patients following dummy treatment. This is known as the placebo effect. There are stories of GPs who, in the past, coloured their routine medicines, and patients who asked specifically for the 'green medicine', claiming that the 'red medicine' had not done them any good! Yet the two might be identical in everything except colour.

We were concerned from the start with how subjective elements could distort the way colds were reported. For example, individual perceptions concerning the frequency of colds suffered were often awry: people might remember two colds in a year but overlook two or three milder attacks. Stalwart characters came to the unit boasting 'I don't get colds doctor, you'll never give me one', but succumbed a few days after receiving intranasal virus drops. It was clear that we had a lot more to learn about the relationship between psychology and colds.

Freedom of choice

In the 1970s more subtle psychological effects were being studied in London. A young psychologist, Richard Totman, wanted to know if 'cognitive dissonance' could be found on the wards of a London hospital. This rather ugly term refers to the mental conflict which arises when there is a contradiction between a person's ideas and beliefs and what actually happens. We were interested in a particular example of this: when our freedom to choose a pill or other treatment results in it doing more good to us than if it is selected for us by a nurse or doctor. Totman studied a ward where patients were given pills for pain relief. Afterwards he recorded how bad the pain had become. He then let some patients choose their pills, whilst the rest had theirs dispensed by the nurse or doctor. In fact all received the same active drug but those who chose their medicine were more improved than those who were given it by the staff.

This experience encouraged him to look for other situations in which the same thing might happen. Almost immediately colds came to mind: most people with colds choose their own treatment, perhaps at a chemist's shop or from the larder or medicine chest at home. And they often swear by the treatment they choose. Is this because cognitive dissonance makes the treatment extra effective? He had to find out.

Totman's problem was the difficulty he foresaw in organising such a study with the erratic and variable colds that occurred naturally in the community.

And it was then that he contacted the CCU to see if he could use our more controlled environment. It was, he thought, an ideal venue in which to carry out a disciplined study. He was right about that, but the results were to raise almost as many questions as answers.

A special programme was set up but proved difficult to design. How would the volunteers react to this new investigation? We could not tell them its real objective until the trial was finished. A number of suggestions were made and it was eventually decided to pretend that the unit was about to test a new drug for colds, though in fact inert capsules of sugar would be used.

Volunteers who consented to take part in the trial were to be divided into three groups: those given the capsule without any option, those who made a positive choice, and those who refused to choose. A number were selected for the first group and the remainder were told they could choose the 'active' drug but would then have their stomach juices sampled by a gastric tube at the end of the trial. This standard but somewhat uncomfortable procedure involves swallowing a fairly large, flexible tube into the stomach, and then withdrawing it – liable to cause a retching sensation. This presented them with a clear choice and, as expected, about half agreed to have the medicine and the rest refused. Then all volunteers were given virus and the results evaluated in the standard way. Of course, we made no request for the passing of gastric tubes and the real reason for the study was explained to everyone.

We had to obtain special permission from the Ethical Committee to do this unusual type of experiment. It was expected that the volunteers who were given capsules 'without the option' and those who refused to choose them would have the usual colds, while those who chose the treatment would fare better. What actually happened was that both those who chose to have the capsules and those who did not had more colds than the comparison group. It was not easy to interpret this. Either the original idea or the study design was wrong—possibly both. We concluded that the volunteers who had spent several days wondering whether to agree to swallow a fat gastric tube had all suffered some form of mental stress. And, whatever they decided in the end, this stress had made them more susceptible to a cold virus infection.

We were used to thinking of resistance to colds as due to immunity of one sort or another but not due to a person's state of mind. We knew, however, that mental changes could produce physical symptoms, like palpitations or stomach upsets, and it might be possible for a cold to alter an individual's skills and mental sharpness. But to believe that the mind could keep a virus at bay did not seem a reasonable hypothesis.

It would have been easy to discard the result on rational grounds: there were problems with the study; the numbers were rather small; the results might have been due to chance; and the whole set-up was so artificial. Even if it showed that psychological stress could change resistance to colds, the type of stress used was unlike anything that was likely to occur in everyday life. But we did not ignore the result. There is an old axiom that the most interesting and important discoveries in research can come from following up the results of an experiment that seems to have gone wrong. It may simply mean it has thrown up something that was not in your mind when you planned it.

Whatever the conclusion, we were determined to pursue it further. So another study was set up along the lines of the previous one. But instead of introducing any artificial stress we asked the volunteers to complete questionnaires concerning any stressful events that had happened at home before they came to the unit. This would tackle the question of whether everyday problems could make them susceptible to colds. There were also questions about their personality.

This second trial once again confirmed an apparent connection between stressful events and increased susceptibility, but again there were some unexpected results. These suggested that introverted subjects had worse symptoms than extroverts and were more likely to be infected. We had expected that psychological factors might make people more sensitive so they would have worse symptoms or describe them in stronger terms. We had not expected to find that their resistance to a virus had changed—especially when the amount of antibodies in their blood had not altered.

The results, though difficult to understand, were published in a paper entitled *Predicting experimental colds in volunteers from different measures of life events*. I believe it to have been a successful study, answering a number of questions but, as so often happens, raising a lot more.

'Not real science'

About this time we had to undergo one of the periodic reviews by which the MRC checked the performance of all its units. A summary of our work over the preceding few years was prepared and circulated to a committee of experts in our field. And then, having studied this, members of the committee, supported by senior administrators, came to Salisbury to discuss our work. Most of this met with their approval—except for the psychology studies. In this respect we were given the impression that these were not considered to be real science, at least not the science we were being supported to do. It was made quite clear that there was to be no more work of this nature.

I could see that such trials might compete with others and reduce some of our scientific output. But the whole idea that the mind could change virus infections, or be changed by them, seemed of crucial importance because it could be applied in so many other aspects of medicine. And we could do rigorous experiments of a type that could not be done in other fields. After all, the unit had been established on the basis that it was ethical to give volunteers a mild virus infection and observe the disease.

In order to resolve the conflict we decided that from then on we would do psychological research as 'piggyback' studies on other experiments. So, in later trials, volunteers in experiments to study virus infection or antiviral drugs were given questionnaires. If it turned out that they were given no virus or drugs their records were ignored. If they were given virus only, sometimes with a dummy drug, then the results of clinical and lab tests were analysed with the psychological data. They did not object and we were able to maintain the double-blind.

At this point Richard Totman decided to change course and leave psychology research. This was in the early 1980s, and there the story might have ended. But fortunately a senior figure in the field—Donald Broadbent—had become interested. After having worked at the MRC Applied Psychology research unit in Cambridge, he had then moved to Oxford University where he had developed some new ideas on how to measure personality and stress and was looking for an opportunity to test these out. He and his wife Margaret—they worked closely as a team—agreed to become the expert arm of another piggyback trial of volunteers inoculated with influenza or cold viruses.

Broadbent introduced his own ideas into the subsequent trials and prepared new questionnaires that reflected his approach. For instance, he identified a characteristic that he called 'obsessionality', though it was not what we usually mean by an obsessional personality. Once again the results showed that personality had an effect on susceptibility to colds and flu. We did not completely understand the mechanics of what was happening but from then on we included a psychology questionnaire in our trials as an aid to assessing whether the volunteers to be given drugs or placebo were equally likely to get colds or influenza.

Do colds affect our performance?

From my earliest days at the unit I had wanted to know whether colds really had an adverse effect on one's ability to perform a task. The world at large seemed to be equally divided between those who thought it did and those who took the opposite view. A pupil at school might be told, 'You've only got a cold, you can still come to lessons'; similarly for those at work. On other occasions the message might be 'If you've got a cold you'd better stay at home until you're over the worst and less of a menace to others!'

There were psychologists at Porton Down, only 10 miles away, but I could not get them interested. Then we heard from a young scientist who was just starting work at the MRC unit at the University of Sussex in Brighton. Dr Andrew (Andy) Smith had trained in applied psychology, obtaining his PhD at University College London at the same time as Totman. From there he moved to Oxford where, as a post-doctoral fellow under Donald Broadbent, he studied the influence of noise on the performance of school children. At Brighton he wanted to look into the effect of minor illnesses as well, and he felt that the CCU would be a good place in which to do this. Its particular advantage to him was that the place was set up for research and he could use the information on symptoms and virus infection that we were collecting routinely from every volunteer.

Andy Smith came to the unit with Donald Broadbent to discuss the idea. He was very keen, well-trained, and based in a good scientific centre—just the sort of person we needed. The disadvantage was that Salisbury was a two-hour drive away. Fortunately, from the early days of the unit we had kept a flat ready for visiting scientists and this we put at his disposal. It meant he could stay on site whenever the length or complexity of an experiment made it difficult for him to return home. Our agreement, quite informal, was that he would start to monitor the way colds affected volunteers moods, skills, and so on. Each day, and sometimes several times a day, he joined the clinical and scientific team which processed daily around the volunteers' huts. I was intrigued at the prospect of what he would turn up.

These experiments could not have been done in earlier years because some of the equipment then in use was too cumbersome to be brought to the huts; and taking the volunteers to the equipment would have compromised the strict isolation that we imposed. But these new tests required very little that was bulky. Some could be done with paper and pencil, some involved sticking pegs in a small peg board, and for others we used an early, portable Sinclair computer. Hand and eye coordination, for example, could be tested by chasing a moving target round the screen with a dot controlled by a little joystick. In other tests the subject responded to simple or complex letters or words by pressing a key. The computer then recorded the results or measured the reaction time, as appropriate.

Our small group of volunteers took to these tests with some enthusiasm. I think they found them a welcome diversion from the routine work of the CCU. We knew that some people would be better than others at doing them, and that their abilities would vary with the time of day. So we used statistical methods that enabled us to compare performances before inoculation with those after the cold developed, while allowing for individual variations. And we did the tests at the same time each day. The results that emerged were most interesting and brought a new dimension to our understanding of the lesser-known effects of the common cold.

Colds do, but not influenza

We observed that the nasal symptoms and signs were most marked in the first quarter of the day, less in the evening, and least in the middle half of the day. Colds interfered with hand and eye coordination skills but influenza infections did not. Conversely the ability to attend to a screen and respond mentally to its message was impaired by influenza but unaffected by colds. So the nature of the problem depended on the virus infection, or rather the type of illness: the same changes were seen when several different viruses were used to produce colds. It was also noticed that the influenza changes were present during the incubation period, when there were no symptoms or signs, and after the volunteer had recovered.

These were fascinating results. The problem was that, whilst we had been able to observe these effects, we still did not know what caused them. In the case of influenza it seemed possible that interferon might be the agent: when we dropped virus into the nose we knew that infected cells there could release interferon into the blood which would then carry it to the brain. But this did not happen with colds. We sought further confirmation by injecting small doses of medicinal interferon into some volunteers, and this did alter performance in much the same way as experimental influenza. However, this was not conclusive since other chemical messengers may play a part in a sick person.

Many tests of performance remained normal throughout colds—for example, the ability to memorise numbers or words for a short period. Andy Smith also used a more difficult test in which the subjects listened to a story being read. After a pause they were asked to recall incidents from the story. The infected subjects remembered everything equally well while the uninfected were good at remembering incidents most relevant to the story line. This indicated an ability to analyse the story as it went along and process it into the memory accordingly. Perhaps this confirms the subjective feeling that one does not get as much out of listening to a lecture with even a mild cold as one does when well.

The idea that colds can have effects in every day life raises a number of questions, particularly with regard to unexpected accidents at work. A lack of attention is frequently the problem but could the primary cause be the effects of a cold? Later in his career, following appointments to posts in the Universities of

Wales at Cardiff and then the University of Bristol, Smith was able to investigate this. Performance tests on volunteers who had caught colds or influenza in the normal way showed changes similar to those seen in Salisbury. Lacking virus-testing facilities, he enlisted the cooperation of interested virologists and again found that cold virus infections and influenza had different effects on performance. Some day we may find out if, and to what extent, accidents are due to unsuspected virus infections. But I know of no current research along those lines.

Stress and colds: an Anglo-American study

Psychologists have their own networks—people in various parts of the world who are working on similar problems. They read each other's papers, attend the same meetings, and visit each other's laboratories and homes. And that is how Andy Smith came to know Dr Sheldon Cohen from Carnegie-Mellon University in Pittsburgh—they had both been working on the effects of noise. They made an interesting pair, quite different in their attitudes and appearance but sharing this common interest. Smith was of medium height, with a fresh complexion and a rather tense manner. Sheldon was taller, pale with a full dark beard, and somewhat more relaxed. However, this calm exterior hid a driving energy every bit as powerful as Smith's.

The department in Pittsburgh had a distinguished research record and was a centre of excellence in computing. Cohen and Smith had talked about the problem of proving that psychological states really did affect diseases and how to measure them properly. Much had been written on the subject but so far nothing had been produced that would stand up to sustained criticism. If such criticism was to be overcome then a different approach was needed. The timing of the psychological tests was important. In early research these had been carried out after an illness, leaving open the possibility that the differences might be the result of the illness, not the cause. The illnesses themselves would also have to be defined in terms of the particular virus infection responsible. And, in order to prove the point more thoroughly, it would be necessary to test much larger numbers—hundreds of patients, not the dozens we had used so far. It was clear that the unit offered an ideal location for tests on such a scale: a study based there would hopefully enable us to confirm and expand on what we had already learnt in our work to date. But it would be a big undertaking and would need money, more people, and close transatlantic cooperation.

Cohen turned out to be an expert in the art of writing grant applications, possibly the most vital of his numerous skills. He had long experience of drafting the many pages of background science, detailed protocols, budgets, and personal details that are required when applying to the US National Institutes of Health for funding. Such people are viewed with respect by their contemporaries and referred to as 'grantsmen'.

Our application took months of letters and revisions, and when the response came it consisted largely of questions to which the referees required answers. We felt that they must want to turn us down, but we were quite mistaken. They thought it likely that we would be successful in showing an effect on colds and wanted us to include further studies to find out how this was produced. We were asked to consider their suggestions as to how this might be done and, to our amazement, they were willing to give us additional money for the extra work, an unlikely reaction had our request been made to a British institution.

The increased funding was a source of considerable encouragement to us. We were now in a position to attack the psychological aspects in a much more comprehensive fashion, rather than with the piecemeal efforts that we had managed so far. But first there were some major practical difficulties to over-come: how to collect the psychological data, combine it with the clinical and laboratory records, and then send it to the USA for analysis. We needed to recruit several new staff who could learn how to administer the question-naires and check the results. Our computers were not powerful enough for the huge database needed to accommodate the results. We had to buy new IBM machines, learn how to use the American software, and then produce discs to send by courier to the USA. They would recheck the figures, sort out any problems, and then begin the number-crunching.

Andy Smith was our key to success in all this, being familiar with all the main components involved: the staff of the unit, the way we worked, the psy-chological tests to be administered, the new computers, and the software.

It was now 1986 and already clear to us that we had a limited time in which to complete the project. News had reached us that the CCU was going to be shut down in 1990. Four years—it was just enough. That was how long it would take to see enough volunteers and complete the bench-work. A quick start was needed and no slippage. Surprisingly this time-constraint only served to increase the morale and enthusiasm of the unit. In the event we completed all the experimental work on time, but still had months of further analyses to complete, followed by the writing of papers.

The road to certainty

Our conclusions began to emerge over the next few years, more certain and more informative than hitherto. Detailed records of each volunteer were sub-jected to powerful statistical computations, throwing up connections that we had missed before. There were 294 people in all, each studied in more detail, taking into account other factors such as the psychological and behavioural characteristics of the individual. They were then infected with a range of viruses—five different strains belonging to three different virus families. And several different measures of mental stress were combined, though separately they all showed the same type of result.

Questionnaires were presented to the volunteers, designed to identify things in life that might stress them: a tendency towards anxiety; times when they felt they were losing control of their lives; situations in which they were unable to cope adequately; and significant events, such as changing a job or losing a close friend or relative. But we recognised that a simple retailing of events would tell only part of the story, and so we tried to find out what these things meant to them. The death of a relative, for example, might cause sorrow at the departure of a loved one or relief at the ending of a difficult relationship.

Assuming that stress had an effect, we also wanted to take the opportunity of testing some ideas about how the effect was produced. For instance was it due to smokers smoking more, or drinkers drinking more, or was it the sort of stress which affected how well people slept or ate? One of these might be the important factor so questions on health practices were included.

Another factor to be taken into consideration was the question of immunity: some volunteers would be immune to a given virus because they had been infected with it earlier and so their blood contained the appropriate antibodies. But our laboratory tests kept us aware of the virus antibody level for each volunteer and so we could allow for this in our statistical calculations.

Volunteers were given a stress score of from 3 to 12 based on the results of the questionnaires. These showed that 47% of those in the most stressed group had colds as compared with 27% in the least stressed group. To our surprise this effect was at least in part due to the fact that stress made them more likely to be infected: laboratory tests showed that 90% of the most stressed were infected, but only 74% of the least stressed. Then more statistical 'control' tests were done to see whether this was due to differences in age, sex, presence of allergy, weight, season of testing, and a number of other variables. Could these be the reason for differences in resistance?

We next sought answers to other questions raised by the computer data. One of these concerned the observation that smokers seem to have worse colds than non-smokers. Our conclusion, unsurprisingly, was that this is probably due to chronic irritation of their airways, making them more prone to coughs and sputum. But it also turned out that they are more likely to catch colds, probably because their immune system is impaired and the airways are damaged.

We did a similar analysis of the effect of drinking on colds, expecting to find that this would also impair resistance, but the opposite effect appeared. Volunteers who did not drink at all, or only rarely, had more colds than those who had one or two drinks a day. Drinks could not be measured very accurately and none of the volunteers were heavy drinkers, so the results have to be treated with caution. But they might imply something akin to the relationship between drinking and heart attacks, namely that moderate drinking is protective as compared with not drinking; although heavy drinking has an adverse effect—sometimes called the J-shaped curve of risk.

The results were analysed further to look for explanations of how stress reduced resistance to colds. The effect was the same whichever of the five viruses had been given—three different rhinoviruses, respiratory syncytial virus, and an influenza virus—and so it looked as though it could be acting through some very general biological defence mechanism, for which we had

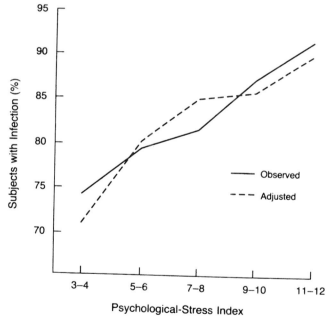

Fig. 10.2 A graph to show the connection between stress and colds. Volunteers who came to the unit were given questionnaires, and from their answers they were graded as to how much stress they had before they came. All were given a cold virus and in the next few days colds were recorded. The results show that those who were more stressed more often developed colds. It can be seen that when the possible contribution of other factors was included, the adjusted results showed exactly the same effects.

failed to test. The total amount of antibodies or specific antiviral antibodies, or the number of white blood cells, had no effect. Items from the general health inquiry—exercise, diet, and sleep—also had no effect. Our analysis showed that smoking and drinking alcohol affected resistance. But when smoking and drinking were used as 'control' variables it was clear that they did not explain the effect of stress.

We had to conclude that the body had some sort of defence mechanism that was weakened by life stress, but we had no way of measuring it except by challenging the subjects with a live virus. There was no evidence that the type of personality was linked to susceptibility—which contradicted some of our previous results. It could have been because the answers to the questions used to assess personality were affected by stress. It could also be that the results were due to chance, which is always a danger when doing small trials. A statistical test may imply the result is 'significant' because there is a probability of one in twenty that it will occur by chance. This much larger study had measured many possibly confusing factors and had been analysed in more detail. It was much less likely that the differences were due to chance. The results confirmed many of the findings of our earlier studies and showed the importance of factors that we had not investigated.

The all-American studies on stress

Our trials had answered questions about resistance to colds and resolved the uncertain results of earlier studies. We would have liked to continue our collaboration with Sheldon Cohen and obtain answers to yet more questions, but this was not possible. The MRC had decided to close the unit at Salisbury.

But Cohen was determined to carry on with common cold trials, and so he organised similar studies in which he collaborated with a group from the Department of Medicine of the University of Virginia in Charlottesville under Doctors Jack Gwaltney and Fred Hayden. They had a long record of expert research, infecting volunteers with their own two 'pet' rhinoviruses, and they were able to test for virus in the nose and for antibodies in the blood. Volunteers were recruited and isolated in a Pittsburgh hotel. Altogether 276 were inoculated with one or other of two rhinoviruses, and the main findings were like those in the Salisbury volunteers. It was a substantial study and extremely important to us: it showed that the experiment could be repeated with similar results, even though the volunteers came from a different society and the virus work was done by a different group using different strains of virus.

Further questions concerning psychological mechanisms were answered by the study. The greatest stresses, it emerged, were caused by 'interpersonal family problems' and 'under- or unemployment', particularly if these lasted for over a month. An interesting new factor uncovered by the Americans was that belonging to various social networks—family, work, social, charity, or religious groups, for example—could reduce the number of colds. Socially isolated subjects were 4.2 times more likely to get a cold when exposed to infection than those with diverse social networks. Unexpectedly, this seemed to be caused by a mechanism other than the effect of stress and did not seem to be due to known factors such as smoking.

The study also showed that people with an introverted personality were 2–3 times more susceptible to colds than the extroverted, which confirmed our earlier findings. Laboratory tests were conducted to see whether the hormones associated with stress, such as those related to adrenalin and cortisone, might explain the effect of stress on colds, but found nothing to support the idea. They came to the same conclusion when they studied a special family of immune cells, known as NK cells, found in the blood and capable of influencing virus infections.

Cohen and his colleagues also did a supplementary trial on volunteers infected with an influenza virus. In this case the virus was adjusted so that all volunteers without antibody became infected. Though all were infected, those with higher stress had more symptoms, while their noses secreted more mucus and contained more of the cytokine IL-6. At the moment it is impossible to interpret these results, but they do suggest that when we get deeper into the problem we will find that chemical messengers like IL-6 are part of the whole picture, perhaps causing the symptoms, responding to virus or to cell damage, or are part of the immune response.

It has taken over two decades to understand this much about the influence of the mind on common colds. When we began, we doubted if there was any effect at all. Now we know that several psychological factors are consistently and predictably linked to differences in susceptibility to colds. However, we suspect that we have not shown how these factors work because we do not understand enough about the biological mechanisms that help us to resist colds. No one has yet tried to prevent colds by reducing stress, and it may be that the best approach would be to block the action of the chemical messengers. The difficulty is that we have no precise idea at the moment as to what they might be.

CHAPTER 11

Hunting for treatments

'We can land a man on the moon, but we can't cure a common cold.' Those involved with research into the common cold are familiar with the jibe. We all hoped that our work would bring a cure nearer, and of course it almost certainly has. But not to the point where something concrete has appeared. In fact no radically new medicines for colds have appeared in the shops since serious scientific research started about a century ago. Not surprisingly, the average person thinks that this is intolerably slow. But that is to misunderstand the nature of the problem and the way in which research and discovery take place.

Novels and popular science books can give the impression that discoveries frequently result from flashes of inspiration that lead straight to conclusive experiments or observations. They can, of course, but only on rare occasions. More usually they occur as a result of long, painstaking research which involves exploring and then escaping from numerous blind alleys before arriving at the hoped-for conclusion. Typically there will be several ideas concerning the answer to a single question. A number of people will do experiments to find which idea is right, and each of them may obtain a different answer. Methods are analysed and modified and more experiments follow until at least a few people get consistent results. Once an idea is proved correct and accepted it will probably raise new questions and the whole process starts again.

Cold research has followed this pattern exactly, except that the possible variations in every aspect of the common cold—its causes, the way it is transmitted, the mechanics of the invasion process, possible methods of prevention, and the distant prospect of treatment—were far more numerous and far more complex than any of us could have imagined. Anyone with the temerity to enter this field soon understands why the common cold has, for so long, been able to defy any attempts to tame it. And it explains why it has been so difficult to progress beyond the initial stage of virus discoveries to a point where there can be a systematic quest for a treatment.

But this sort of thing has happened before. The bacterial causes of pneumonia were discovered in the late nineteenth century, yet specific treatment with serum, soon replaced by sulfonamides (a group of drugs suitable for the treatment of a number of conditions) did not appear until the 1930s. Viruses were discovered later, and by 1960 some of the important ones were known and could be handled quite easily in the laboratory. Only then could a focused search for specific treatments begin. We were to find it was an area that would not yield answers easily.

Work begins again

Antibacterial drugs were in use by 1960. Some of them, like sulfonamide, were synthesised by chemists; and others, like penicillin and streptomycin, were made by fungi. But most of these had no effect on viruses. In fact we were able to use penicillin and streptomycin in all our tissue cultures to keep bacteria at bay while the viruses were growing. Chemical compounds capable of stopping viruses generally did so at concentrations which damaged cells and so were toxic to animals. This is not surprising since viruses use the cell's own components to build new viruses. Anything that stopped this process probably did so by interfering with the machinery of the cells in which they were replicating. One exception was a synthetic drug that was active against the tubercle bacillus but also stopped pox viruses growing. This led to an anti-smallpox drug, Marboran (isatin beta thiosemi-carbazone). Successful tests against the disease in India in the 1960s showed that here was at least one drug which could stop a virus growing and damaging tissues and might benefit patients. However, this was an isolated case.

Over half a century earlier the pioneering German scientist, Paul Ehrlich (1854–1915), put forward the idea that bacteria might be attacked by molecules which stuck to them specifically, like dyes, and did not damage human cells. The discovery of antibiotics showed that he was right. But it looked as though it would be a lot more difficult to do the same sort of thing with viruses. And the more that was understood about the virology of colds the more obvious these difficulties became. In the absence of any clear-cut path ahead people sometimes followed up unlikely clues or tried short-cuts on the road to developing treatments, hoping that they might stumble on something. This was understandable since valuable drugs had been found in the past when a keen observer noted something unexpected and followed it up. For example, a seventeenth-century English physician, William Wittering, noticed that some patients with dropsy (swelling of the legs with fluid) improved when given some country remedies and showed that all the effective medicines contained foxglove. He did not understand the mechanism, but the active principle, digitalis, is still in use to treat heart failure.

But taking a flyer like this succeeds only rarely, disappointment being the more usual outcome. For instance, in the mid-twentieth century, antihistamine drugs were being developed and would dramatically stop the nasal symptoms of patients with hay fever. The sneezing and nose running were so like those of patients with colds that it seemed possible they would have a beneficial effect on them as well. An experiment at the unit to check this out found that the drugs had no such effect on a cold induced with one of our 'pedigree' viruses; and other researchers in the UK, USA, and elsewhere came to the same conclusion. In colds, the nose is made to run by something other than histamine.

Just a spoonful of vitamin

Vitamin C, or ascorbic acid, was the subject of a much larger study later on and the cause of some controversy. It all started when chemists in a laboratory in Switzerland developed the habit of taking spoonfuls of it off the shelf whenever they felt a cold coming on, and they were sure that this stopped it developing. Such claims from people with a scientific background were bound to raise hopes that vitamin C might offer an effective treatment. The idea was given extra credence when it was promoted by the American, Linus Pauling, a Nobel Prize winner and an outstanding physical chemist, who recommended consuming 12 grams a day. This, he calculated, was the amount swallowed by our near biological relatives, the gorillas. Who could fail to be impressed by such a recommendation!

Unfortunately these claims ignored one rather large area of doubt which attaches to all these supposed cures or treatments for the common cold. The cold symptoms which we experience from time to time frequently fade away overnight without causing us any further discomfort, and without our taking any steps to treat them. We have all had a slight case of the snuffles, a nose or throat irritation, or a pricking of the eyes, only to have these things go by the next day. It simply means that we are harbouring a virus that has attacked us in the past: our bodies quickly recognise its structure and immediately bring the immune system into action. Such occasions probably exceed by quite a margin the number of times we actually succumb to a cold. But if we have taken some treatment at the time then it will appear that this has been responsible for the disappearance of the symptoms.

In spite of these doubts vitamin C became the vogue, and it was even proposed that huge doses should be supplied on the National Health Service. Anything capable of having such a beneficial effect on the nation's health and economic productivity was clearly worth considering, and even spending some money on. But could it really stop a cold?

Studies were conducted at the unit by Georgina (Neena) Walker, a lively and enthusiastic young doctor from Glasgow with an interest in infectious diseases and a desire to be involved in research. She tried to show that large amounts of ascorbic acid added to a tissue culture would stop viruses growing—but to no effect. We decided to try it out on human colds. Our volunteers were inoculated with cold viruses, one half being given three grams of vitamin C each day—more than that caused side-effects—while the other half were given dummy vitamin tablets. But there was no discernable difference between the two groups, both having exactly the same number and type of colds.

Dr Pauling wrote from California to say that he was not impressed. He pointed out that we should give the vitamins just as the cold symptoms start and not before the virus drops. We had been giving the vitamin early so as to give it the best chance of showing any effect. We tried the experiment again, ensuring this was taken into account, but the result was the same. Pauling then said, quite correctly, that with our relatively small number of cases we could not exclude the possibility of a modest effect which, by chance, had not shown up. And anyway we had not studied 'real colds' but only the artificial imitations used at the unit.

We could not meet this challenge at Salisbury, but by this time we were linked with the epidemiology department at the Clinical Research Centre at Harrow. Dr Tom Meade there organised a trial at several centres, including Salisbury, in which a thousand participants took certain tablets when they felt a cold coming on. When the code was broken it turned out that exactly the same proportion of colds developed in those given vitamin C as in those given a dummy. I do not recall getting an answer from Dr Pauling after I wrote to tell him the result.

Although our results were so uniformly negative we had to draw our conclusions very carefully, and so we could not say honestly that ascorbic acid had no effect. We could only say that in a study capable of detecting a small effect, and at the dose used and with well-nourished subjects, no benefit was detected; and we concluded that it would not be worth using clinically to help against colds. It is interesting that a number of studies have now been done worldwide and these were recently analysed as a group—a so-called meta-analysis. It was concluded that there may in fact be a small beneficial effect. However, this does not alter my view that the proper use of vitamin C is to prevent deficiency and treat scurvy. It may benefit colds, if given in massive doses, but these can also produce harmful effects.

Why not attack the bacteria?

Many people still believed that bacteria helped to produce colds, perhaps by adding to the damage done by a virus, as happened in animal diseases. So why not try to treat colds by attacking the bacteria? Colleagues repeated the vaccine treatments that had been tried some years before, but with increased controls, to see what effect there might be. It had been found that if bacteria from the nose were cultured and a specific vaccine was made for individuals, then colds were slightly milder. But the work was complex, the improvement slight, and the series of injections inevitably caused some discomfort. We concluded that the whole thing was not worthwhile.

It was rather easier to use vaccines made from standard laboratory bacteria. These were tried repeatedly but in the end it was agreed that a very thorough study in the USA was right and that they did no good at all. In spite of this, vaccines given by mouth were still being sold up to the 1970s. We studied one of these oral vaccines to see if it could stimulate antibodies in the nose when injections would not. But months of work produced no evidence of any difference in the colds of those who swallowed killed-bacteria and those who took a dummy fluid.

People still believed that there was a 'bacterial phase' in the development of colds and that they would be milder if we eliminated this phase by giving patients antibiotics. It seemed a plausible idea but early work on this possibility was not encouraging. Trials have continued, using different drugs in varying circumstances. A recent survey by the Cochrane Collaboration, a group concerned with the ethical use of drugs, finally selected nine which were really well done but still showed no benefit.

Of course colds can be followed by recognised bacterial infections such as pneumonia and pus in the middle ear, and these need proper antibacterial treatment. But it should be noted that giving antibiotics in virus infections does not reduce the number of bacterial illnesses that follow; it just makes it likely that when they occur they will be due to drug-resistant bacteria and therefore difficult to treat. The wrong use of drugs in colds is a significant problem at the present time and is discussed later.

Specific anti-viral treatment: influenza

In spite of the difficulties, there were some early successes in the hunt for drugs against respiratory viruses. The discovery of amantadine and later drugs shows how research can detect and develop a drug that works in patients. The story begins in the early 1960s when virologists and chemists at the Dupont company in the USA suspected that molecules with amino groups (an atom of nitrogen and two of hydrogen) attached might stop the influenza virus growing. They tested a number and found one in which the amino group was attached to a rigid 'cage' of carbon atoms, and this protected mice from drops containing enough influenza A virus to kill them with pneumonia.

When given to humans it was well tolerated except for giving some mild shakiness and wakefulness—the molecule is a bit like Benzedrine. So it was tested in volunteers who were exposed to the virus in the form of nasal drops or spray and then given the drug regularly by mouth. The results were somewhat variable. A small trial at the unit produced negative results, but trials elsewhere showed that it did prevent disease. Later tests suggested that it would be beneficial even if given after the symptoms had started. Numerous trials followed confirming that it was effective in adults and children living in the community and elderly persons in retirement homes. In due course it was licensed and could be prescribed for the prevention and treatment of influenza A.

It is normal in drug research that when a molecule is found with some useful properties it is used as a 'lead' compound. This means that chemists take the molecule as a starting point, adding to or subtracting from it at various points, hoping that this will 'lead' them to a molecule with more valuable properties—more active, easier to give, and so on. So chemists then took amantadine as a lead compound and synthesised numbers of other molecules in an attempt to develop different properties that would make it more useful. One molecule called spiroamantadine was tested in volunteers at Salisbury and was effective, but not sufficiently improved to be marketed. Another, called rimantadine, has been extensively studied in the USA and Eastern Europe and is in clinical use. ICI in the UK developed a molecule with a nine-member (nonane) carbon ring which, in careful tests in animals at their laboratories and in volunteers at Salisbury, seemed to offer a real improvement. But the high costs of developing it as a drug and its rather limited, and therefore less profitable use, made it an uneconomic development. The company decided they would use their money to develop more promising compounds for other conditions.

There are two interesting tailpieces to this story. One concerns an unexpected use for amantadine. It was noticed that when given as a treatment for influenza to patients with Parkinson's disease it also improved their nervous system symptoms; and this improvement was maintained even when there was no influenza about.

The other development could be of great benefit to future influenza sufferers. The influenza virus contains a neuraminidase, an enzyme that enables the particle to get into and out of cells. It does this by cutting away sugar molecules to which a protein on the surface of the virus sticks. As a result the virus can penetrate through the sugars to reach the inside of the cell and, similarly, escape from the layers of sugar when it is time to move on and attack other cells. During the 1990s in Australia the neuraminidase was purified and then crystallised. The crystals were subjected to X-rays and, from the scattering of the rays, the researchers could work out the shape and composition of the molecule's active centre, the part that actually splits off the sugar: it looked like a tiny propeller. This was fundamental knowledge concerning the virus, and the key they were looking for. They could now calculate how a molecule with atoms arranged in a particular way would interact with the atoms forming the propeller. From these results they could then predict a small number of molecules that would bind tightly to the centre and prevent it splitting off sugars. Under these conditions the virus would be unable to find its way into a cell or to escape. It offered the potential for developing a truly novel, anti-influenza drug.

They were correct in this assumption. The molecules did what was expected of them and formed the vital components in anti-influenza drugs developed by Glaxo-Wellcome in the UK and Gilead and Roche in the USA. Both drugs prevent and treat influenza A and B infections.

Any drugs against cold viruses?

Influenza viruses, because of their small number and greater predictability, lent themselves to this logical form of research and offered much greater opportunities for success in the battle to bring them under control. But our problem was the cold virus, or rather the cold viruses in all their vast number and variety. Drug development was moving ahead fast, as we have seen in the fight against influenza. But back at the CCU in the 1960s the future was much less certain.

Following our success in growing the rhinoviruses, we were interested in finding a treatment for similar viruses and had just started working with the coxsackievirus A21, mentioned earlier. It was like a rhinovirus, caused colds, but was much easier to deal with. Our intention was to use this in an experiment with one of a number of so-called steroidal antibiotics that had been studied in Denmark. We had found that this particular antibiotic would stop virus growth in the laboratory and was known to be safe for human use. However, when we gave it to our volunteers it failed to prevent infection or illness. It transpired that there was quite enough in the blood to stop virus growth, but it was not getting through into the nasal secretion. That taught us an important lesson. Rhinoviruses, as their name suggests, only attack the nose; and so even active drugs would only work if they entered the circulation and then reached the nose. The best way to ensure this was to introduce the drug using nose drops or sprays.

Jennifer Doggett, another product of the CCU grapevine, was the young woman who carried out this important work. Having taken a degree in microbiology at Bristol University she began work in a hospital bacteriology laboratory in the Midlands, but a friend from university days, already employed at the CCU, recommended that she came to join her. Jennifer applied as soon as a vacancy was announced and found the friendly, family atmosphere, as well as the science of the unit, much to her liking. She did excellent work on a variety of projects and was one of the number who also benefited from the informal education provided by Christopher Andrewes' morning walks. This clearly made an impression for, after marriage and the raising of a family, she became warden of a nearby downland nature reserve, well-known for its orchids.

Later in the 1960s we were joined by Paul Beare, first mentioned in Chapter 8. His first project was a search for antiviral drugs. He and his colleagues had been studying inhibitors of influenza neuraminidase, though without the sophisticated methods mentioned above. The idea was good in principle and, by routine screening, they found two molecules that blocked the enzyme and stopped virus multiplication. They were not toxic and seemed ideal material for practical trials. One of the attractions of working with us was the avail-

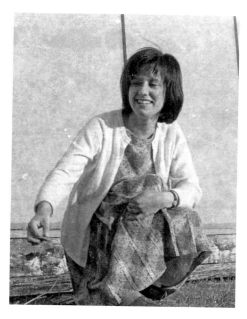

Fig. 11.1 Jennifer Doggett. (From Jennifer Acornley.)

ability of our volunteers and the possibility of testing these compounds in humans. The drugs were given well before the virus and throughout the subsequent infection so they would have the best possible chance of success. And under these conditions there seemed to be a very weak benefit.

Further research showed that the compounds actually attacked the virus particle directly but that one of them, 2054, also stopped a typical common cold rhinovirus from multiplying. They were again tested in volunteers but without the desired result. It seemed they were not sufficiently potent to be worked on further, and so the chemists were asked to make related compounds that might function better. But there was no improvement on the two molecules we had tested and we decided to bring that particular project to a close.

Sylvia Reed, who was introduced in Chapter 9, came to us about this time, her arrival coinciding with claims by workers in the USA that they could prevent colds with some recently discovered molecules. Once more we were being presented with that elusive prospect, a cold cure. She decided to investigate. Sadly, the claims turned out to be unfounded. It was a familiar ending to this type of investigation but that did not make it any less disappointing at the time. Of course such studies were an essential part of our work, and it was of great help to potential manufacturers to know that a particular drug would not be effective in colds.

But some of those drugs were tested against other viruses in other situations and found to be effective. For example one of these, Ribavirin, has proved to be life-saving in some very lethal virus infections such as Lassa fever.

Sylvia Reed conducted a number of valuable studies while at the CCU and was a model for others in her careful approach to research. In some of her work she was assisted by overseas students, and for them the clinical studies, laboratory work, and their contact with her were all of long-term benefit.

Interferon—a natural treatment

Interferon, already mentioned a number of times, must now take centre stage. First identified in 1957, it was not until 1973 that we were able to report on its potential as a means of preventing colds. Some important early work was done on this at the unit and it later had a great impact on the search for antiviral treatments in general. The key man initially was Alick Isaacs. One of two bright twins who qualified in medicine in Glasgow, he decided from the outset that, unlike his brother, he did not want to treat patients. Laboratory work on infectious disease was what interested him. I met him first in

Sheffield when he was working on influenza viruses for Charles Stuart-Harris and I was a young house physician. He was lean, animated, and seemed to get a lot of fun out of life. We shared a common interest in music, but my earliest recollections are of him quizzing me about what I thought was happening in virus 'interference'. What process was going on, he wondered, when one virus, already in a cell, stopped a second virus from growing?

He went to Australia and I met him next when he returned to work at the World Influenza Centre at the NIMR, Mill Hill. He was studying how viruses spread around the world and how they behaved in the laboratory. It was there, with Jean Lindenmann from Switzerland, that he probed what had happened when one of his experiments on growing virus in chicken cells 'went wrong'. He discovered that viruses inside cells can stimulate them to produce a protein that can then enter other cells and inhibit the growth of viruses there. He named the protein interferon. It was a nice simple name quite unlike the usual chemical terms. But then, as he pointed out, why should physicists have all the good names such as electron?

Isaacs' fertile mind was full of ideas about interferon: how it might work, whether it helped people recover from infections, and whether it could be used, like penicillin, to treat virus infections. Many scientists thought it was a rather uninteresting finding and that some of his experiments might be flawed. Someone in the USA even went so far as to re-christen the substance 'misinterpreton'. But the MRC did not share this lack of faith and set up a small committee of its own staff and representatives of three pharmaceutical laboratories. It was chaired by Isaacs and was known as the Scientific Committee on Interferon. Meeting at intervals, it studied how to produce interferon and purify, test, store, and use it to prevent and treat infections.

There were problems. For one thing the substance was incredibly active and there was very little of it in experimental samples. It was also very difficult to concentrate and purify. We were one of the laboratories involved, who were working together in an informal and friendly way sending each other materials and results whenever it seemed these might help. However, as it was planned to patent the drug, there were limitations on who we informed and what we published prior to any patent application. This was because there were fears that, without such precautions, the country might end up paying royalties to foreign firms for the product of a 'British' discovery—as was felt to have happened in the case of penicillin.

Interferon had no sooner been discovered in London than we found that we already had some down in Salisbury. In trying to explain why cultures of calf kidney cells might recover from influenza virus infection we found that they were producing interferon. But when we tested our calf interferon in chicken cells and Alick's chick interferon in calf cells it became clear that interferons might not work in cells of a different species. A study was immediately set up and this showed that interferons from human and monkey cells would protect cells of either species, but chicken interferon would not. So we would have to use a human or monkey interferon in order to treat human disease.

It was now clear that each species produces its own type of interferon; but it then transpired that, in each case, this could take a variety of forms. For example interferon-alpha, the name given to the interferon produced by many human cells when exposed to viruses, appears in at least half a dozen different versions. And fibroblast cells (basic cells of human, fibrous connective tissue), when exposed to virus or nucleic acid, produce another form of interferon which, though similar, is sufficiently different to deserve a new name, interferon-beta. Cells of the immune system, when activated, turn out a quite distinct molecule called interferon-gamma. This can also make cells resistant to virus infection, but its main role is as a chemical messenger that communicates with other cells of the immune system.

Glaxo was, at that time, making polio vaccine using monkey kidney cells, so it adapted the process to make interferon. It was a crude preparation and not very active, but in a joint study among the collaborators we showed that if injected into human skin it would stop the 'take' of smallpox vaccine. This enabled us to report in 1962 that laboratory-made interferon would stop infection in intact human tissue. It was time to try it out on a more natural human infection.

We needed to make a large amount of monkey kidney interferon and then spray it into the noses of our volunteers to see if it prevented infection and experimental colds. It took several years to produce a suitable batch but it did not protect against colds. This was quite a blow, for we had begun to think that the process had real possibilities. Our best guess was that we had not used enough interferon, but we had now exhausted our entire stock and, for the time being, could not conduct any more experiments. We needed a better source of supply—perhaps human interferon.

A Pacific mould offers hope

Interest in interferon had grown substantially by the mid-1960s, and in the USA there was an informal programme for the exchange of information between workers in the field. International meetings were discussing the subject and papers were appearing in scientific journals. While I was in New York

I met Richard Shope, the friend of Andrewes first mentioned in Chapter 3, who shared our interest in virus research. He told me that, during the war while serving with the US navy in the Pacific, he noticed some mould growing on a photograph of his wife which he kept in his cabin. Remembering how penicillin had been discovered he carefully preserved some of it with a view to studying it more closely in peacetime. If it led to the discovery of a new drug he planned to call it helenine after his wife, Helen.

Once hostilities were over he returned to work at the Rockefeller Institute and found that fluids in which the mould had grown did in fact protect mice from virus infections of the nervous system. This observation was followed up by scientists at Merck Laboratories in New Jersey, and they reported that this was because the fluids contained a double-stranded nucleic acid which stimulated the animals to produce large amounts of interferon.

These findings attracted the interest of a number of investigators, among them the scientists of G. D. Searle in the UK who decided to enter the field using a process which seemed to offer a good chance of success. By this time it had become relatively easy to grow human fibroblast cells in the laboratory and so they planned to stimulate these to produce human interferon. We agreed that when the material was produced and tested it would be tried out in volunteers at Salisbury. It was nearly 1980 before the study was completed and again, to our intense disappointment, there was no benefit. Apparently the interferon had lost activity while being stored or manipulated.

While all this was going on we were doing experiments with interferon from human blood. It all stemmed from the work of Kari Cantell in Helsinki. He had taken human white cells from the Finnish Red Cross, stimulated them with a parainfluenza virus and found that, in the right conditions, they poured out large amounts of interferon. This was partly purified and given to patients, particularly for treatment of cancers. Cantell generously offered to let us have some of his material which, at that time, was a substantial proportion of all the interferon in the world. This was partly purified and prepared by Glaxo in the UK and tested for safety in primates by Smith Kline in Belgium.

One of our visiting scientists in 1972 was Tom Merigan, an outstanding worker from Stanford University in California, who showed that influenza B was also sensitive to inhibition by interferon in test-tube culture and tried it on a group of volunteers to see if it would prevent infection. Volunteers given dummy interferon were also inoculated for comparison. The only immediate effect was to make the incubation period a little longer. He was not deterred as he had seen something like this when trying to protect chickens against infection. So the study proceeded and he set out to use the interferon to prevent rhinovirus colds and infection in the volunteers. Not wishing to err on the side of giving them too little, Merigan made round after round of the flats until he had given the volunteers 39 sprays of interferon or placebo between the day before inoculation and the time when illness was expected. We then waited expectantly for him to plot out the results, our excitement rising as it became clear that some of the treated people had been partly protected from virus attack. We could see that the differences were statistically significant and not likely to arise by chance.

The impact worldwide was considerable. A number of groups were encouraged to carry out their own experiments with interferon, to find better ways of using it, and to look for other drugs. But everyone was handicapped by its scarcity.

During the 1970s we tried compounds from ICI in Britain, Rhone Poulenc in France, and Ciba Geigy in Switzerland, which certainly stopped virus growth in the test tube. But when they were tried out in experiments, like those done with interferon, none had any measurable clinical effect, though they seemed to reduce the growth of virus a little.

Other workers, and particularly Maurice Hilleman of Merck whom I knew from the time when we had worked in adjacent labs in New York, said that the best thing would be to get the body to make its own interferon. In other words to use the new interferon inducers as medicines instead of interferon itself. His firm had developed a synthetic product that worked as well as mould extracts. We continued our work on interferon itself, but cooperated with Beecham Laboratories in Britain to try out this alternative idea.

The Beecham interest arose through one of their advisers, Ernst Chain, well known as a joint Nobel Prize winner with Alexander Fleming and Howard Florey for his work on penicillin. He thought that there might be an antiviral, as well as an antibacterial, drug hidden in *Penicillium* mould. Working at London University, but jointly with Beecham, he found a virus in the mould containing a double-stranded nucleic acid that induced interferon in the laboratory. It took several years to develop as a drug and worked well in protecting mice, but less well in monkeys. It was time to see if it worked in our volunteers.

Chosen to carry out the clinical part of these studies was an able young visitor to the Clinical Research Centre, Dr F. Y. (Freddy) Aoki. Born in Canada of immigrant Japanese parents, he had graduated in medicine there and come to England as a visiting worker to study antiviral treatment. He set up and ran an early trial on modern, purified rabies virus vaccines and then joined us to do these trials of the interferon inducer in volunteers. Afterwards he joined the University Department of Infectious Diseases in Winnipeg and has since played a key role in international trials of new anti-influenza drugs.

The interferon inducer was tested against cold virus infections at Salisbury and found to induce irritation and nasal symptoms in the human nose; and at just about the dosage that was needed to protect the nose against infection. Similar findings had been obtained independently with synthetic inducers in the USA.

The experiments with interferon showed that an antiviral sprayed up the nose could block a virus growing there and prevent the symptoms of infection. This encouraged us and scientists in the pharmaceutical laboratories to continue screening development programmes to find a convenient small molecule that would do the same and be easier to produce. Several firms had found molecules that stopped virus growth at lower concentrations than we had seen before, and they were willing to produce the extra amounts and do the safety tests that would be needed before we tested them in volunteers.

But we wanted to find a better way of producing and purifying human interferon, though we had no really new or promising ideas. The director of the NIMR, Sir Peter Medawar, decided to help us by arranging a small brainstorming session in which we were joined by some outstanding people from the Laboratory of Molecular Biology at Cambridge. If sheer brain-power could solve the problem then we should have been well on the way to doing so, for amongst the participants were two Nobel Prize winners, Medawar himself and Francis Crick. The session went well, but the only conclusion we reached was that we should look more deeply into the way interferon is synthesised in human cells.

We were not aware of it then, but our problem was already well on the way to being solved in another, very new and very different area of science.

Genetic engineering to the rescue

New DNA techniques were now extending the boundaries of biotechnology and permitting a much deeper understanding of the life processes. Genetic engineering was very much the coming thing in the late 1970s—not in the sense of cloning animals but as a means of producing specific materials relatively cheaply and in large quantities. We mentioned earlier how it was possible to introduce DNA into a bacterium which would then produce more DNA—known as DNA cloning. But methods were also developed to introduce DNA into bacterial and other cells in such a way that the DNA would instruct the cell to synthesise the particular protein that it specified—known as DNA expression. These techniques are known as recombinant DNA technology. Once the rules had been established it became possible to harvest large quantities of protein. Insulin was immediately recognised as a likely candidate and is now produced in this way. The hope was that interferon would also be amenable to the process. But was there a danger that new bacteria might be created that would pour out harmful molecules?

This was exciting stuff, and not a little frightening: no one was quite sure where it was all leading. The risks needed to be assessed, and initially a voluntary moratorium on all such experiments was declared. I remember a meeting on the issues involved chaired by Sir Robert Williams, then head of the Public Health Laboratory Service. Discussion assumed a rather depressing tone as it focused on the harm these experiments could do if they went wrong. But I pointed out that if we did get the work going successfully there would be enormous benefits for patients, and I mentioned the possibilities of synthesising valuable medicines such as insulin and interferon. 'But how long would that take?', I was asked. I thought for a while and then replied: 'About ten years.' It was not my most accurate prediction: about two years later we began using human interferon produced by genetic engineering.

We were fortunate that several groups wanted to produce human interferon in this new way. In fact there was quite a race on. For one thing they wanted to prove that a molecule could be made so accurately that it would have all the properties of the natural product. Interferon was a medium-sized protein and it would be particularly impressive to produce it in the cells of a bacterium, like the bowel organism *Escherichia coli*, and show it was specifically active in human cells. There was also a real hunger for the molecule, particularly among those who wished to use it as adjuvant treatment for cancers and people like us who wanted to investigate it as an antiviral. The first group to clone, sequence, and produce human interferon-alpha was led by Charles Weissmann in Switzerland. They had a link with the American pharmaceutical company Schering-Plough, who quickly set up a process to produce material for clinical trials.

Our trials followed the usual pattern. But they had to be documented even more elaborately than before, partly because Schering-Plough wanted to have data for a licence application, and partly because the amount of detail now demanded in any clinical trial was increasing steadily. We were able to use more interferon than ever before and the results showed that the number of colds and the amount of rhinovirus shed were markedly reduced.

During the same period there was another crucial experiment based on new molecular techniques. For this we collaborated again with Kari Cantell. He provided leucocyte—white blood cell—interferon as before, although we knew that most of the material in the fluid was not interferon but contaminating cellular material. We wondered whether it could be something, unrecognised in the mixture, that actually protected the volunteers. This time we were able to expose the mixture to a monoclonal antibody against human interferon. It was extremely specific and would bind only to interferon. So the rest of the mixture was washed away and the interferon was released as a pure protein from the antibody. When given to volunteers this protected them just as well as standard preparations.

We had successfully demonstrated that both interferon made in bacteria, and that made in human cells and fully purified, would protect against cold viruses. It followed that the protection must be due to the interferon molecule itself.

Later in the 1980s we tested other genetically engineered interferons against rhinoviruses and showed that other products were effective, including interferon-beta. Interferon-alpha was also active against influenza and corona viruses. However interferon-gamma, which is chemically and biologically quite distinct, did not protect well. Indeed, it may have added to the inflammatory response.

All our work so far suggested that interferon had some potential, but was it a practical proposition for the treatment of colds, and were there simpler and more economical ways of using it, rather than the multiple doses of our original trials? So we worked our way systematically through the possible regimes and found that, once colds had developed, administering interferon had no effect. If it was to have any chance of success then it had to be given during the early stages of the incubation period. This presented an almost impossible scenario because it meant that it would have to be administered before anyone knew that a cold was imminent.

Several groups, including ones in America and Australia, repeated some of our experiments and confirmed the results. They then went on to see if these could be applied to dealing with colds in the community. Selected families were given interferon sprays which members could use on themselves when someone in the household developed a cold. These studies were very carefully done with a placebo group accompanied by full clinical and virus records. It seemed that the number of colds caught was slightly reduced, and this was due to reduced rhinovirus infection. But there was no measurable effect on infection with any other viruses.

Other studies showed that after subjects had been taking regular interferon by nasal spray for a week or two they developed stuffiness and other nasal symptoms. These were shown to be due to infiltration of the nasal membrane by white cells. The inflammation then disappeared when the treatment was stopped. These so-called toxic effects of interferon have been overcome when it has been used for the treatment of chronic conditions like cancer and hepatitis, but not in the case of upper respiratory virus infections.

I believe that our mission to explore the use of interferon against colds, conducted over many years, was as detailed and comprehensive as possible. It seemed to offer the possibility of leading towards some sort of cold cure, but its inherent problems could not be overcome. We reluctantly concluded that, for the reasons mentioned above, it would not be possible to market interferon as a preventive or treatment for colds.

Molecules that home in on viruses

Antiviral treatment in the form of virus-binding molecules became a fascinating area of study, and one in which we saw some prospect of success. It all started with a series of apparently quite unconnected lines of research and ended with the focus on a small area on the outside of a virus particle and the successful prevention of experimental colds.

Wellcome Research in England were trying to find active antiviral molecules by screening various foods and natural products, like oranges. Some anti-rhinovirus activity was observed, and in due course the active ingredient was identified as a flavan. Wellcome then synthesised a particularly active derivative (dichloroflavan) which, at the time, had the highest active antiviral activity in the test tube of any known molecule, and was non-toxic. Thus it had powerful effects on rhinoviruses but none on animal or human cells.

Nippon Roche, the Japanese section of Hoffmann La Roche, was looking for new treatments in Chinese traditional remedies. In one of these, a tea recommended for the treatment of colds, they discovered an anti-rhinovirus molecule, known as chalcone, that was non-toxic and would inactivate the virus particle.

Over the years the laboratories of Janssen in Belgium had been remarkably successful at synthesising and developing a number of valuable and effective drugs, and in the course of this had built up a large bank of compound molecules. It occurred to them that amongst these they might find an antiviral cold cure. A systematic screening programme was set up and they eventually found activity in a molecule which had been produced while searching for a sedative or tranquilliser. Derivatives were made and these proved to be active against rhinoviruses, though not equally against all serotypes.

Sterling Winthrop in the USA was interested in a material called actidione, which had been extracted from the liquors from which streptomycin had been produced. This was found to be active against polioviruses, binding to, and then inactivating them. The Sterling Winthrop group made a large number of molecules of the same general shape and found that by interchanging certain atoms it could increase or decrease the ability of the molecules to bind to the virus. Amongst these were some molecules that would bind to rhinoviruses which, as I mentioned earlier, are similar in biological terms to polioviruses, and the other enteroviruses.

These were molecules of more than passing interest and we determined to investigate them in our laboratory and establish their antiviral properties. But we needed someone to handle the project. It was our good fortune to find a person who was more than qualified for the task we had in mind.

The man from Kuwait

Widad al-Nakib, introduced in Chapter 6, was born in Basra where his father was a well-known local doctor and one-time chairman of the British Medical Association in the Middle East. Educated first in English language schools in Alexandria, Widad came to England for his secondary education and took A levels from a small boarding school near Banbury in Oxfordshire. He was the only one taking biology and, since there was no teacher conversant with the subject, he largely taught himself. From there he went to Trinity College Dublin, where he studied microbiology, moving to London for his PhD. But his particular interest was medical virology.

At St Thomas' hospital he introduced leading-edge, immunological methods for the study of rubella (German measles). Then, having married, he returned to Kuwait, where his parents had since moved, and played a key role in starting the new medical school there. But he had no intention of becoming a desk-bound administrator at his early age and decided to return to London for a sabbatical year at the bench. It was while working on a virus using molecular methods that he heard through the grapevine that we were looking for someone to work in our laboratory and with volunteers. He thought this was too good an opportunity to miss and immediately offered his services. We were only too happy to take on such an ideal man— and one, furthermore, who did not need an MRC salary!

At the bench in Salisbury he found that all the new molecules were highly active against rhinoviruses. However, they were disappointing in volunteer trials. Dichloroflavan, it transpired, was not absorbed from the gut, but had to be reformulated so that it would be taken up and enter the bloodstream. But it did not enter the secretions of the nose, and we believed this to be essential if it was going to affect virus growth. It was formulated yet again and given directly into the nose but still did not prevent colds or affect the rhinovirus infection.

The antiviral chalcone discovered in the Japanese tea provided a similar experience. This time a chemical derivative was made which was absorbed into the blood and then converted into the active molecule in the body. But it did not pass from the blood into the nose. Again an intranasal formulation was needed, but this, too, was ineffective.

Finally, the Janssen drug was studied. This was formulated with a chemical that had been developed by the firm for use in the food industry and probably worked by folding itself round the individual drug molecules. Treated in this way they were almost soluble and, if given as a nasal spray, stopped virus shedding and colds. More accurately, it delayed them, for there was some evidence that if the drug spray was stopped the virus could start to multiply again.

Basic work on the drugs ran in parallel with trials. Rhinovirus type 14 was a favourite virus for study. Its RNA sequence was known and it had been crystallised. Michael Rossman at Purdue University in the USA had worked out

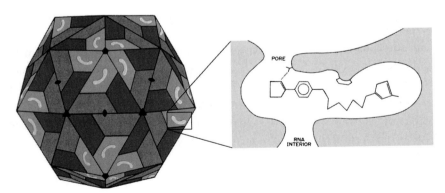

Fig. 11.2 A diagram of a rhinovirus particle showing the pattern of triangular facets on the surface capsid proteins. In the surface there is a groove or canyon that is part of the mechanism by which the virus enters the cell and 'uncoats'. There is a cleft at the bottom of this area which a capsid-binding drug molecule has entered. This prevents the virus uncoating, releasing its RNA, and so infecting the cell (Based on work of M. Rossman).

the structure of the particle by X-ray crystallography. The group at Sterling Winthrop then soaked a crystal in one of its compounds and crystallography revealed that it had fitted itself into a cleft on the surface of the particle which is believed to be concerned with the virus getting into the cell. This could explain why these compounds, as a group, make viruses non-infectious but make the particle resistant to heat as well; and why, if the compound is removed with a solvent, the virus becomes infectious again. The viruses mutate rather easily and become resistant to the drugs; and in some cases when this happens it has been shown that the atoms around the cleft have been rearranged: one of the amino acids forming a part of the cleft has been exchanged for one of a different shape. Presumably the drug no longer fits into the slot. The drug also has less effect on some types of rhinoviruses than on others—the cleft is lined with rather different amino acids. This drug resistance could make it difficult to use the Janssen molecule clinically although, in certain cases, the problem can be overcome by using combinations of drugs.

Koen Andreis in Belgium also did a lot of work on the sensitivity of different serotypes to various related molecules. He looked for something that would be highly potent against a wide range of viruses and had some success. However, the main difficulty in developing the drug is that it has no effect if given after symptoms have appeared. When tested on families in Charlottesville in Virginia it gave no observable benefit. We concluded that, in this type of infection, by the time symptoms appear, key cells have been invaded; and the effects of this are not reversed if the virus is held back by interferons or a synthetic drug.

In other diseases, such as tuberculosis and AIDS, it is now the custom to prescribe a cocktail of drugs, as this increases the potency of their effect and reduces the appearance of drug-resistant mutants. This can be readily shown in laboratory experiments on rhinoviruses, and we made a tentative effort to apply it to volunteers by treating them with combinations of a rather weak antiviral drug, enviroxime, and an interferon. Unfortunately no benefit was seen.

Are better drug treatments possible?

People treat their colds with a mixture of methods, some traditional, some based on pharmaceutical chemistry. And, as we have seen, some of these are reasonable while others are not. Much of our work at the CCU was designed to increase our understanding of the causes of colds

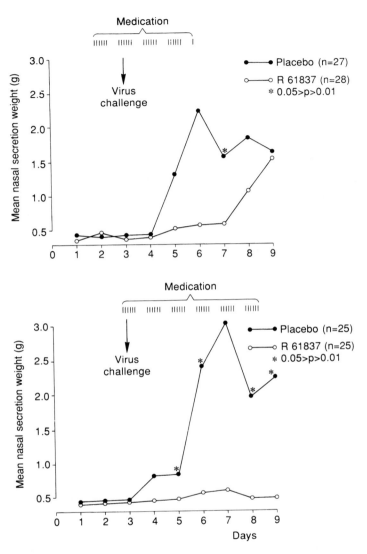

Fig. 11.3 A graph showing the effect of regular intranasal sprays of a capsid-binding drug on groups of volunteers infected with a rhinovirus. Those given sprays without drug developed colds after the usual two or three days. Those given drug showed no increase of symptoms. The stars show days on which the reduction in secretion was statistically significant – i.e. unlikely to occur by chance, see Table 7.2.

to the point where we could hinder the progress of a virus infection. The unspoken assumption was that, as in the case of, say, pneumonia or typhoid fever, the disease would then rapidly subside and the patient would feel well again.

Our failure to affect the disease with powerful antiviral treatments like interferon or capsid-binding drugs could mean that we have still not found sufficiently powerful molecules, or that we have not delivered them to the places where the infection is focused. But we did try a variety of approaches, so attacking the virus at this stage may be ineffective. After all, in healthy adults we know that the body's defences deal very quickly and efficiently with the invaders. Only in rare cases does the virus spread widely.

Perhaps we should leave the attack on the virus to the immune system. Recent work on how to deal with acute gastroenteritis indicates that the patient is not helped by antibiotic treatment, even if a sensitive bacterium is the cause. What does help is to correct the loss of fluid and salts from the bowel by giving a suitable solution by mouth, and this is now the foundation of good management throughout the world. It could well be time to correct the assumption on which the search for antiviral drug began and start to look seriously for ways of correcting symptoms like nasal blockage and discharge. I remember being told that this was *only* symptomatic treatment, with the inference that it was inadequate and second-rate. But it is the symptoms which cause the discomfort. Removing these must surely be desirable. And our immune system can quietly get on with eliminating the virus. The less we know about it, the better we will feel.

It so happens that the present is a very good time at which to begin research of this sort. We now have detailed knowledge of the various viruses that start the disease process, what they do to the cells they infect, and how the immune and other defence systems of the body respond. We already know some of the possible chemical messengers which may switch on these mechanisms.

Before the unit closed we took a first step in this direction. We tested a molecule that, to some extent, blocked the action of one of the possible messengers, bradykinin, known to cause irritation of the airways. It had just been shown that bradykinin is released into the nose during a cold and, conversely, if it is sprayed into the nose of a healthy person it induces symptoms like those of a cold. Either because the messenger was not very important or because the block was not effective there was no measurable effect, but at least it was a first step down this path.

It is just possible that continued research might produce such a drug. We could then block the messengers or their targets on the cells, reducing the level of discomfort we might otherwise feel, and without delaying our recovery from illness. Achieving this would have a big impact on our attitude towards the common cold, reversing our centuries-old impotence in the face of its attacks. As we have pointed out, it is only rarely that the virus attack itself causes us any problem—our immune system usually deals with this most efficiently. But the ability to remove the symptoms could transform our lives—at sleep, at work, or at play.

Epilogue: The end of the road?

The CCU closed in 1990. It had been given a long run, far longer than anyone had anticipated at the outset. And, in spite of some disappointments, I believe it largely achieved what it set out to do. It identified the causes of the common cold, established how it is transmitted, analysed its distribution and significance on an international scale, looked at its interaction with other diseases, investigated the psychological implications, studied and demythologised much of its folklore, and even searched for a cure. In short, it provided a scientific basis for most aspects of the disease.

When the CCU opened in 1946 its main purpose was to find out what caused colds, how they were transmitted, and what their effects were. The idea of finding a cure would have seemed very remote at that stage, since our knowledge of the common cold was rudimentary in the extreme, and much of that was based on false assumptions. Our understanding was transformed by the work which followed, and we were able to follow in detail the progress of a cold from the first moment of infection right up to its final stages and eventual elimination. But of course it is the failure to find a cure which has hit most strongly upon the public consciousness. Why, people will ask, in this age of advanced science, do we appear to have got nowhere in combating this age-old affliction?

The truth is that we have made enormous progress, though it has needed detailed research in many centres. Knowing its causes, the mechanics of how it is caught and its variety of forms is a very significant advance. But it is this variety which is at the heart of the problem. What had appeared to be a single disease capable of a single solution turns out to be something of unimagined complexity for which there is no straightforward answer.

Perhaps one of the common cold's main problems is that it is not sufficiently virulent. 'Familiarity breeds contempt' is a proverb which could have been devised expressly to describe our attitude towards it. If it was more frequently life-threatening, like smallpox, polio, yellow fever, and AIDS, which are all caused by viruses, then perhaps research into its effects and a possible cure might have begun much earlier, been more widespread, and been maintained over a longer period. Even so I find it remarkable that so much patience, time, and effort was put into the work of the CCU, particularly in view of the competing demands of other research projects in a time of financial stringency and in the face of so many disappointments. As Shakespeare said so felicitously, there is a tide in the affairs of men, and maybe we were just fortunate in catching such a tide: a moment when a nation had just emerged from a terrible war, with fear as to its outcome replaced by a new spirit of optimism. We can only hope that such a tide will return one day and provide the conditions in which the research can be brought to a conclusion.

The appearance of AIDS, more than anything else, concentrated minds on the practice and understanding of infectious disease medicine. However, it also meant that common acute respiratory infections were seen as less important compared with this threat of a worldwide, lethal plague. It was inevitable that huge funds would be diverted for research into such a dreadful disease, and work on AIDS has shown that if enormous resources are directed at a problem then the chances of success are substantially increased. After some 15 years of intensive work the HAART (highly active anti-retrovirus treatment) regimes were developed, which seem to arrest the progress of the disease and its complications. Admittedly the virus cannot be eliminated, and the regimes are cumbersome and very expensive. But the amount of scientific progress is impressive. Part of the reason seems to be the amount of relevant research that has been done at all levels, from molecular studies of the virus to the pathology of the disease processes in humans and animals.

Meanwhile, respiratory infections continue worldwide and have significant health and economic effects. Our concerns are not restricted simply to the common cold. Asthma, for example, a disease which was almost unknown a hundred years ago, is now highly prevalent, and we need to learn more about the role of viruses in precipitating attacks. And there are many other areas. Medical research priorities change from year to year, but I hope it will soon be possible to return to a concerted attack on the common cold. As I have already said, there are some promising lines of research which could lead to a better control of the virus or our response to it. Perhaps then we can reduce the heavy load of mild or moderate ill health that is borne by all sections of society.

Further reading

In this section we provide the reader with signposts to publications that will give more detail on the events, or background to our story, old ideas about colds, the work of the CCU, the debate about the use of volunteers, and so on.

Andrewes, C. H. (1965). *The common cold*. Weidenfeld and Nicholson, London.

Andrewes, C. H. (1973). *In pursuit of the common cold*. William Heinemann, London.

Beecher, H. K. (1966). Ethics and clinical research. *New England Journal of Medicine*, **274**, 1354–60.

Bull, D. (1992). The common cold a historical perspective. Unpublished dissertation for BSc History of Medicine. University of London.

Bynum, W. F. (1994). *Science and the practice of medicine in the nineteenth century*. Cambridge University Press.

Chadwick, J. and Mann, W. (1950). *The medical works of Hippocrates*. Blackwell, Oxford.

Cliff, A., Haggett, P., and Smallman-Raynor, M. (2000). *Island epidemics*. Oxford University Press, New York.

Gerard, J. (1633). *The herbal*. Reprinted by Dover publications, New York, 1975.

Kruse, W. (1914). Die Erreger von Husten und Schnupfen. *Muenchener medizinischer Wochenschrift*, **61**, 1547.

Landsborough Thomson, A. (1987). *Half a century of medical research*. Vols 1 and 2. Medical Research Council, London.

Lowbury, E. (1990). *APOLLO: an anthology of poems by doctor poets*. Keynes Press, BMA House, London.

Medical Research Council (1964). Responsibility in investigations on human subjects. *British Medical Journal*, **ii**, 178–80.

Mellanby, K. (1972). *Human guinea pigs* (2nd edn). E. W. Classey, Hampton, Middlesex.

Pappworth, M. H. (1967). *Human guinea pigs: experimentation on man*. Penguin, Harmondsworth, England.

Payne, A. M.-M. (1953). The influenza programme of WHO. *Bulletin of the World Health Organisation*, **8**, 755–74.

Royal College of Physicians of London (1984). *Guidelines on the practice of ethical committees in medical research*. Royal College of Physicians, London.

Tansey, E. M., *et al.* (1998). The MRC Common Cold Unit. In *Witnesses to twentieth century medicine* (ed. E. M. Tansey and L. A. Reynolds), pp. 209–68. Vol. 2. Wellcome Trust, London.

Thompson, K. R. (1990). *Harvard hospital and its volunteers*. Danny Howell Books, Warminster.

Waterson, A. P. and Wilkinson, L. (1978). *An introduction to the history of virology.* Cambridge University Press.

Wesley, J. (1770). *Primitive physick or an easy and natural method of curing most diseases.* William Pine, Bristol.

Whitelock, O., Furness, F. N., Stahl, F. S., and Sturgeon, P. A. (ed.) (1957). *Cellular biology nucleic acids and viruses.* Special Publications of the New York Academy of Sciences, New York.

This section gives a few references to papers and reviews which report key discoveries or review them in scientific terms. Of course, it is possible for readers who have access to scientific textbooks or their associated CD-ROMs, or to the Internet, to obtain many more references, including current publications.

Beare, A. S. and Reed, S. E. (1977). The study of antiviral compounds in volunteers. In *Chemoprophylaxis and virus infections of the respiratory tract* (ed. J. S. Oxford), pp. 27–56. CRC Press, Cleveland, Ohio.

Beeson, P. and McNair Scott, T. F. (1942). Clinical, epidemiological, and experimental observations on an acute myalgia of the neck and shoulders; its possible relation to certain cases of generalised fibrositis. *Proceedings of the Royal Society of Medicine,* **35**, 733–40.

Buckland, F. E., Bynoe, M. L., and Tyrrell, D. A. J. (1965). Experiments on the spread of colds II: studies in volunteers with coxsackievirus A21. *Journal of Hygiene (Cambridge),* 63, 327–43.

Chanock, R. M., Roizman, B., and Myers, R. (1957). Recovery from infants with respiratory illness of a virus related to chimpanzee coryza agent (CCA). I. Isolation, properties, and characterisation. *American Journal of Hygiene,* **66**, 281–90.

Chanock, R. M., Parrott, R. H., Cook, M. K., *et al.* (1958). Newly recognized myxoviruses from children with respiratory disease. *New England Journal of Medicine,* **258**, 207–13.

Cohen, S. and Rodrigues, M. (2001). Stress, viral respiratory infections, and asthma. In *Asthma and respiratory infection* (ed. D. P. Skoner), pp. 193–208. Marcel Dekker, New York.

Crawford, D. H. (2000). *The invisible enemy.* Oxford University Press.

Dick, E. C., Jennings, L. C., Mink, K. A., Wartgow, C. P., and Inhorn, S. L. (1987). Aerosol transmission of rhinovirus colds. *Journal of Infectious Diseases,* **156**, 442–8.

Dingle, J. H., Badger, G. F., and Jordan, W. S. Jr (1964). *Illness in the home: a study of 25 000 illnesses in a group of Cleveland families.* Western Reserve University, Cleveland, Ohio.

Hamre, D. and Procknow, J. J. (1966). A new virus isolated from the human respiratory tract. *Proceedings of the Society for Experimental Biology and Medicine,* **121**, 190–3.

Hilleman, M. R. and Werner, J. B. (1954). Recovery of new agent from patients with acute respiratory illness. *Proceedings of the Society of Experimental Biology and Medicine*, **85**, 183–8.

Holmes, M. J. and Allen, T. R. (1973). Viral respiratory disease in isolated communities: a review. *British Antarctic Survey Bulletin*, **35**, 23–31.

Kapikian, A. Z., James, H. D., Kelly, S. J., *et al.* (1969). Isolation from man of 'avian infectious bronchitis-like' viruses (coronaviruses) similar to 229E virus, with some epidemiological observations. *Journal of Infectious Diseases*, **119**, 282–90.

Lidwell, O. M. and Somerville, T. (1951). Observations on the incidence and distribution of the common cold in a rural community during 1948 and 1949. *Journal of Hygiene (Cambridge)*, **49**, 365–81.

Myint, S. and Taylor-Robinson, D. (ed.) (1996). *Viral and other infections of the human respiratory tract*. Chapman and Hall, London.

Rowe, W. P., Huebner, R. J., Gilmore, L. K., Parrott, R. H., and Ward, T. G. (1953). Isolation of cytopathogenic agents from human adenoids undergoing degeneration in tissue culture. *Proceedings of the Society for Experimental Biology and Medicine*, **84**, 570–3.

Thomson, D. and Thomson, R. (1932). *The common cold: annals of the Pickett-Thomson Research Laboratory*. Vol. 8. Baillière, Tindall and Cox, London.

Tyrrell, D. A. J. (1965). *Common colds and related diseases*. Arnold, London.

Tyrrell, D. A. J. and Bynoe, M. L. (1965). Cultivation of a novel type of common cold virus, in organ cultures. *British Medical Journal*, **1**, 1467–70.

Tyrrell, D. A. J. and Parsons, R. (1960). Some virus isolations from common colds. III Cytopathic effects in tissue cultures. *Lancet*, **1**, 239–42.

Index